Clara Barton's Civil War

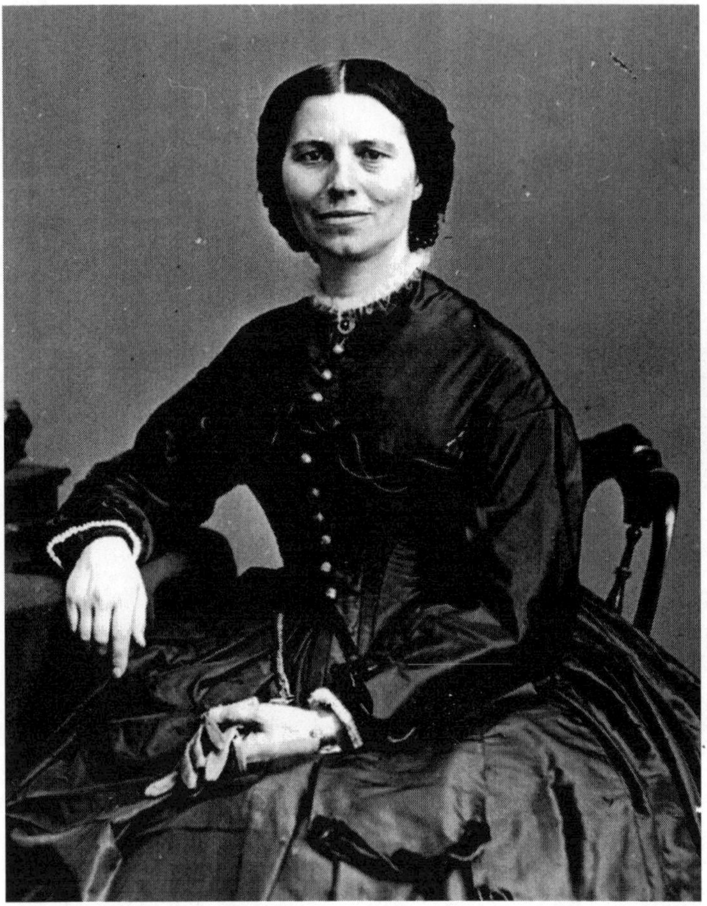

CLARA BARTON'S CIVIL WAR

BETWEEN BULLET AND HOSPITAL

DONALD C. PFANZ

WESTHOLME
Yardley

Facing title page: Clara Barton, c. 1865, photographed by Matthew Brady. (*Library of Congress*)

First Westholme Paperback 2022

Westholme Publishing, LLC
904 Edgewood Road
Yardley, Pennsylvania 19067
Visit our Web site at www.westholmepublishing.com

ISBN: 978-1-59416-389-0
Also available as an eBook.

Printed in the United States of America.

To my late wife, Betty,
The sweetest, most courageous nurse of them all.

My business is staunching blood, and feeding fainting men—my post, the open field, between bullet and hospital.

—Clara Barton to Thaddeus Meighan, 1863

Contents

Preface

As a historian at Fredericksburg and Spotsylvania County Battlefields Memorial National Military Park, I first became interested in Clara Barton while reading Stephen Oates's *A Woman of Valor*, a book that describes her actions as a Civil War nurse. Oates portrays Barton as a heroine of mythical proportions, standing up to corrupt and incompetent officials, overcoming obstacles that would have defeated others, and saving countless lives by her resourcefulness and determination. At first, I accepted the stories he recounted at face value, but as their number multiplied I grew suspicious. There were too many coincidences, too much drama. Something wasn't quite right. Where did the author get his information? I began checking Oates's footnotes and to my astonishment discovered that the source for most of his heroic tales was Clara Barton herself. That set off alarm bells in my mind. Then and there, I decided to dig out the original sources, peel away the self-manufactured legend, and determine for myself what she really did during the war.

That was not as easy as it first appeared. As the park's staff historian, I had read thousands of letters and memoirs written by Union soldiers, *and not one of them* so much as mentioned Barton. I thought this odd given her heroic conduct and the fact that she was one of a very small number of women serving at the front. Surgeon J. Franklin Dyer was in charge of the Lacy House hospital in

Fredericksburg where Barton worked for more than two weeks in December 1862, yet his only comment about Barton came eight months later in a letter to his wife, and that reference was hardly flattering. General Marsena Patrick did not mention Barton at all. She encountered the Army of the Potomac's provost marshal in town on the day of the battle and gives a stirring account of their meeting. Yet in his diary Patrick is silent about the encounter. He obviously forgot about it or did not think it worth recording. Even more remarkable, Barton does not have a single reference in *War of the Rebellion: A Compilation of the Official Records of the Union and Confederate Armies*, the 128-volume set of official correspondence generated by the war, nor in the equally exhaustive *Medical and Surgical History of the War of the Rebellion*. Even the official history of the 21st Massachusetts, her pet regiment, mentions her just once and that in a very general sort of way. As one of just a few women working among thousands of men, Barton should have stood out. That she did not is remarkable and perhaps significant, for it suggests that her role on the battlefield may not have been as important as she later claimed.

Of the few accounts written by others about Clara Barton's experiences at Fredericksburg, most appear to be spurious. For instance, Miss H. P. Cleaves, in a speech delivered shortly after Barton's death, told the story of an episode that supposedly occurred near Fredericksburg in which a regiment of soldiers formed a line across a stream and knelt down on one knee forming a human bridge across which Barton walked. Cleaves insisted that Barton herself told her this story. While that may be true, it does not make it any less absurd.[1] Only slightly more believable is an article by a Captain Joseph Hamilton that appeared in the magazine *Woman's Home Companion*. In it, the mysterious officer extolled Barton's heroism at Fredericksburg. A close reading of the article, however, exposes numerous errors and shows it to be based in large part on Barton's own speeches.[2]

Even Linus Brockett, in his otherwise admirable book *Light and Shadows of the Great Rebellion*, yielded to a measure of gullibility when he recorded that Union soldiers, in the midst of the battle, brought Barton a carpet for her quarters that they had stolen from a private house. In a moral tale worthy of Parson Weems, he has Barton insisting that the soldiers return the purloined item. E. R. Hanson, in his 1884 book *Our Woman Workers: Biographical Sketches of Women Eminent in the Universalist Church for Literary, Philanthropic and Christian Work*, goes even further, asserting that Barton refused to leave the beleaguered town until she had seen the furniture and valuables of the dwellings used deposited safely in the buildings, where they could be reclaimed by their owners upon their return.[3]

Another source frequently quoted is an 1887 letter by Honora Connors, a woman seeking a government pension for her services as a Civil War nurse. Connors wrote to Barton on February 15, 1897, soliciting her assistance in obtaining the pension. In the letter, Connors recalled serving with Barton in 1864 at hospitals located in Fredericksburg's courthouse and Catholic church. "I remember that you used to wear when you came in to visit the sick soldiers, a blue dress and a white cap; and that you used to sing 'Rally round the flag, boys!' and that Gen. Barlow's wife used to come down to the hospital sometimes with you." Unfortunately, Connors appears to have confused Barton with someone else. Barton was in Fredericksburg fewer than sixty hours in 1864, and thanks to her diary we know much about whom she met and what she did there. The diary says nothing about her meeting Arabella Barlow nor of her visiting either the courthouse or the Catholic church. While she might have made brief stops at those places, she could not have served alongside Connors for a significant period of time as the letter suggests.[4]

Also open to question are some of the statements made about Barton's actions on other battlefields. A few are demonstrably false, such as surgeon James Dunn's assertion that Barton visited his field hospitals at Cedar Mountain and Second Manassas or that she was still at Antietam when he left that place four days after the battle. Likewise without foundation is a statement that Barton supposedly made to Lenora B. Halsted that she helped administer chloroform in the operating room at the Poffenberger farm after all but one of the surgeons had fled. Other stories are merely improbable, such as that of a veteran who approached Barton after a postwar speech and informed her that she had treated him on not one, but three, different fields of battle: Fairfax Station, Fredericksburg, and Bermuda Hundred. While the statement *might* be true, it is highly unlikely as few regiments fought in all three places. Moreover, the soldier told Barton that his leg had been "shattered" at Fredericksburg and yet he maintained that he was able to return to duty, something likewise improbable.[5]

So how does a historian get at the truth when his subject is so firmly steeped in legend? The key is to revaluate the source material; in this case, primarily Barton's own writings. Were they written at the time or in later years? Was she writing for herself only or for an audience? When writing about her own deeds was she a reliable witness or prone to exaggeration? Can what she wrote be confirmed? If not, is it plausible? Such were the guideposts I used in pursuing my research for this book. The result, I hope, is a more realistic but no less remarkable account of Clara Barton's Civil War.

1

The Angel of the Battlefield

"SINEWS OF STEEL AND NERVES OF IRON"

Certain names in American history are recognized by virtually everyone: George Washington, Benjamin Franklin, and Abraham Lincoln, to name but a few. Clara Barton also falls into that category. Every schoolchild in America knows her name—or should. As a nurse, she was perhaps the most famous woman to emerge from the Civil War. But she did not stop there. Almost singlehandedly, she persuaded the United States Congress to ratify the Geneva Convention, an international treaty regulating the treatment of sick and wounded soldiers on the battlefield. At the same time, she founded the American Red Cross, an organization that to this day provides relief to victims of war and natural disaster. She is an American heroine and rightly so. But how much do we really know about her?

We should know a great deal. Since her death in 1912, dozens of books and articles have been written about Clara Barton's life. However, most are long on adulation and short on critical analysis. The Civil War years are a case in point. During the war she kept a diary, wrote occasional letters for publication, and corresponded with family and friends. Afterward, she traveled throughout the

North delivering speeches about her wartime service. Much of what we know about her in those years comes from these sources. Unfortunately, most of Barton's biographers fail to differentiate between her writings, accepting them all at face value. The diary entries, written for her eyes only and on the days when events actually transpired, can be trusted. The letters that she wrote to newspapers and to private correspondents, while frequently melodramatic in tone, are generally reliable too. However, her speeches are another matter altogether. Writing years after the events, Barton dramatized them in order to appeal to audiences who had paid good money to hear her speak and wanted to hear a compelling story.

Barton's own story started on a farm in south-central Massachusetts. Her father, Stephen, was an enterprising New Englander and a solid citizen of the community, a "calm, sound, reasonable high-toned moral man," in his daughter's judgment. He worked as a farmer, businessman, and sawmill owner and served as an officer in the local militia. At times, he was a selectman for his town, and in 1836 he was a representative on the Massachusetts General Court. As a young man, Stephen had served as a noncommissioned officer under "Mad Anthony" Wayne in the Northwest Indian War, and in later years he whiled away cold New England nights regaling his young daughter with tales of his military adventures. His stories fired the girl's imagination and instilled in her a keen sense of patriotism. A tomboy at heart, she dreamed of becoming a soldier herself and of one day serving her country as her father had done.[1]

Stephen showed Clara a tenderness that she did not find in her mother. Sarah Stone was a quarrelsome woman with a quick temper, whom Clara thought "both *nervy* and *nervous*." She was difficult to please and swore when angry. Sarah was always up before the dawn, squeezing two days' work into a single day. She was a sensible, no-nonsense woman who taught her daughter the virtues of industry and thrift but gave her little in the way of love or encouragement. When Sarah died, in 1851, Clara refused to dress in black, telling an acquaintance that she did not mourn because she did not grieve. Perhaps owing to her mother's difficult personality, she developed

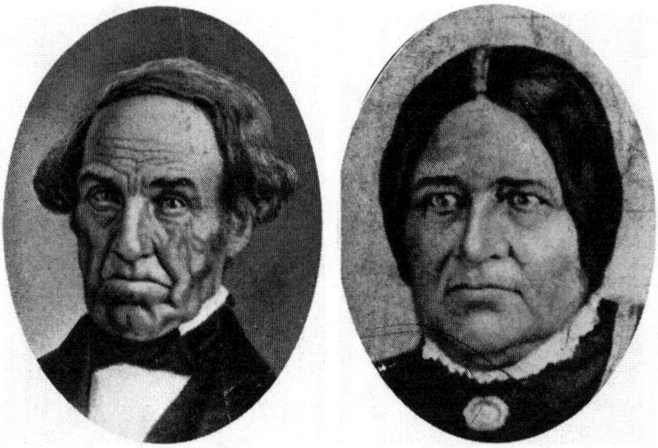

Clara's parents, Stephen and Sarah Stone Barton (*Library of Congress*)

into what she later described as a "diffident, timid, non-committal" child, "afraid of giving trouble." If she went through this phase, she outgrew it.[2]

Clara was born on Christmas Day, 1821, near North Oxford, Massachusetts, a small town situated roughly eight miles south of Worcester. The modest white frame house where she grew up still stands. Christened Clarissa Harlowe Barton, she eventually shortened her name to simply Clara. At the time she entered the world, her parents already had two sons, Stephen, Jr., and David, and two daughters, Dolly and Sally, all of whom had been born more than ten years earlier.[3] Clara was small for her age, had close-cropped hair, and spoke so softly that it was sometimes hard to understand her. From the start, she displayed a sensitive nature. She once fainted at the sight of an ox being slaughtered and afterward did not eat meat, if she could help it. It was a strange reaction for a woman who in later years voluntarily surrounded herself with bloodshed and death.[4]

When Clara was still a young girl, her father sold the homestead to his sons and purchased a 300–acre farm for himself. The four older children continued to reside on the old farm, while Clara and her parents moved to the new place. As she grew older, Clara helped with many of the outdoor chores there, such as cultivating the garden, milking the cows, and tending the farm's many ducks, hens, turkeys, and geese. Her greatest joy, however, was feeding and grooming the horses. From a young age she loved to ride, and when she was ten her father bought her her own horse.[5] By then, she was already an experienced rider. When she was five, her brother David had taught her to ride by throwing her on the back of a colt and, with Clara holding fast to the mane, set off with her in "wild glee" across the fields. She enjoyed it thoroughly. Late in life she wrote, "To this day, my seat on a saddle or on the back of a horse is as secure and tireless as in a rocking chair, and far more pleasurable."[6]

David was Clara's favorite brother. When she was still young, he had suffered a bad fall and for two years was an invalid. Throughout that time, Clara remained constantly at his bedside, administering medicine, applying leeches, and tending to his every need. "I could not be taken away from him except by compulsion," she later wrote, "and he was unhappy until my return." She did not realize it at the time, but she had found her calling.[7]

Nursing was not then a profession, however, and as Clara became a young woman, it appeared that she would be a schoolteacher, one of the few vocations open to her sex. She was well educated herself, having attended both public schools and a boarding school at different times in her life. When not under the tutelage of professional teachers, her siblings had guided her studies.[8] By the age of sixteen she was ready to begin teaching. In 1838, she taught forty students in a one-room schoolhouse near her home. Four of the boys were nearly as old as her and promised to be trouble; however, Barton quickly gained their respect by besting them in sports. "When they found that I was as agile and as strong as themselves, that my throw was as sure and as straight as theirs, and that if they won a game it was because I permitted it, their respect knew no bounds," she recalled. "No courtesy within their knowledge was neglected."[9] She had proved herself superior to men and in doing so gained their respect. It is a theme that appears over and over again in her writings.

But such tactics did not always work. The following year, while teaching in the nearby town of Charlton, Barton came up against a gang of insolent and unruly boys who delighted in disrupting her class. She finally had enough. Calling their leader to the front of the room, she pulled out a whip and proceeded to lash the young man until he apologized to the class for his actions. After that, neither he nor the others gave her any more trouble. "I had learnt what discipline meant," she later wrote, "and it was for all time as far as that school was concerned." Barton could be just as tough with prospective employers. When offered a teaching position in Oxford, she refused because the school board offered her less money than they would have accorded a man. "I may sometimes be willing to teach for nothing," she told them, "but if paid at all, I shall never do a man's work for less than a man's pay." The board members acceded to her demands and gave her the salary she deserved.[10]

For several years, Barton moved from school to school, gaining valuable experience. After taking off a year to study at New York's Clinton Liberal Institute, she tried her hand at teaching in New Jersey. In Bordentown, she started a free school for indigent children. The school attracted just six students on its first day, but as word of her teaching spread, attendance swelled to upwards of 600. In fact, the school was so successful that town trustees voted to expand the building to eight rooms and hired a superintendent and seven additional teachers to staff it. Barton expected the trustees to offer her the superintendent's job, and when it went to a man instead she was understandably upset—particularly when she learned that the he would be earning $600 a year, more than twice her own salary. She left the school a short time later.[11]

Bordentown left a sour taste in Barton's mouth for teaching, and in 1854 she moved to Washington, D.C., to become a copyist at the United States Patent Office, making transcripts of original records. She did well at the job and soon took on the more responsible work of abridging original papers and preparing records for publication. Financially, she thrived. "She was an excellent chirographer, with a clear head for business," remembered a friend, "and was paid by the piece and not by the month"; consequently, "she made money fast." Very fast. In an era when wage earners typically did not make more than $500 a year, Barton pulled in $1,400. She was an outspoken Republican, however, and in 1856, when Democrat James Buchanan was elected president, she found herself out of a job. She only regained her position four years later, after Abraham Lincoln took office.[12]

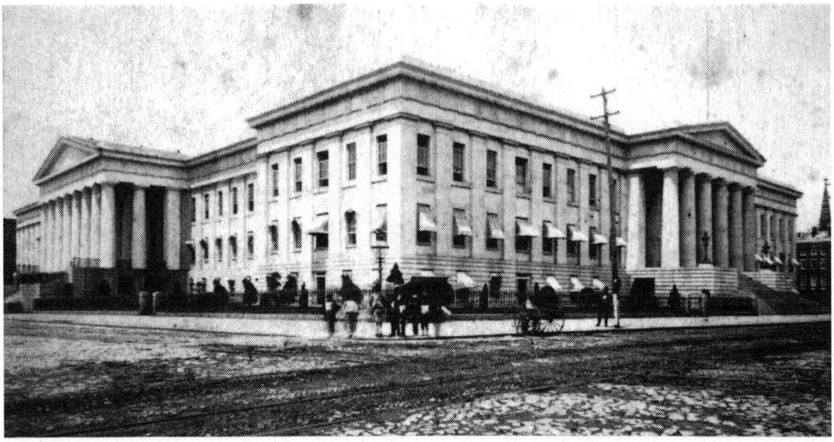

The United States Patent Office in 1860. (*Library of Congress*)

Barton was still at the Patent Office in April 1861 when Southerners fired on Fort Sumter, inaugurating the Civil War. Rumors of the bombardment swept through the capital, creating a frenzy of excitement. In a letter to a cousin, Barton wrote that Washington was divided in sentiment and "growing warlike." On one street corner recruiters were enlisting men to fight for the Union, while on another pro-Southern speakers were telling listeners that the Union no longer existed and that the "Constitution was a mere pretense, and our government a myth." Barton at this point in her life was not an abolitionist, but she was a staunch Unionist and such words angered her. For months she had listened to secessionist harangues, and she was fed up with them. "From the bottom of my heart I pray that the thing may be tested," she seethed. "May the business be taken in hand and *proved*, not '*if*,' we have a Government, but *that* we have one, and those [who] have revelled in its liberties, and fed and fattened on its bounties be taught to respect it." Like the rest of the country, she was growing warlike.[13]

What up to now had been largely a war of words soon turned into a war of bullets. Three days after Confederate troops raised their flag over Fort Sumter, the 6th Massachusetts Militia started south to defend Washington. As it passed through Baltimore, Southern sympathizers assailed the regiment with stones, bricks, and even small-arms fire. Four soldiers died in the riot, and another three dozen suffered injury. The 6th Massachusetts responded by firing into the crowd, killing twelve civilians before hurrying on to Washington. Sick and wounded members of the regiment sought care at the Washington Infirmary, while the rest set up temporary quarters in the Capitol. Barton felt a strong connection with the troops from her native state. After paying a visit to those confined in the hospital, she proceeded to the Capitol to visit friends and acquaintances there. One of the soldiers had just received a copy of their hometown newspaper, the *Worcester Spy*, and someone suggested that Barton read it to them. She gladly obliged, reading one article after another from the vice president's chair. "You would have smiled to see *me* and my *audience* in the Senate Chamber of the U.S.," she related to a friend. "Oh! but it was better attention than I have been accustomed to see there in the old time."[14] The comradery she experienced there had a profound effect on Barton. "From that hour," wrote an early biographer, "she identified herself with the soldiers in their risks and sufferings."[15]

At that particular moment the soldiers' greatest source of suffering was a lack of supplies. The men had lost their baggage in the Baltimore fracas and reached Washington with little more than the clothes on their backs. Some had "not a cotton shirt and many of them not even a pocket handkerchief," Barton reported. She gave the soldiers the few supplies she had with her and then hurried home to gather up more. By the end of the day, she and others had filled a large market basket with all manner of items, including serving utensils, thread, needles, thimbles, scissors, pins, buttons, strings, salves, and tallow.[16] She continued to bring food, sewing supplies, and other small items to the soldiers over the coming months, at the same time acting as "mother and sister" to those who were ill. When the people of Massachusetts learned of her activities, wrote historian Linus Brockett, they began shipping her boxes of "clothing, lint, bandages, cordials, preserved fruits, liquors, and the like" for the men. In order to store the large influx of goods she received, she had to rent no fewer than three warehouses.[17]

While Union troops gathered in Washington to defend the capital, additional states broke away from the Union and joined the

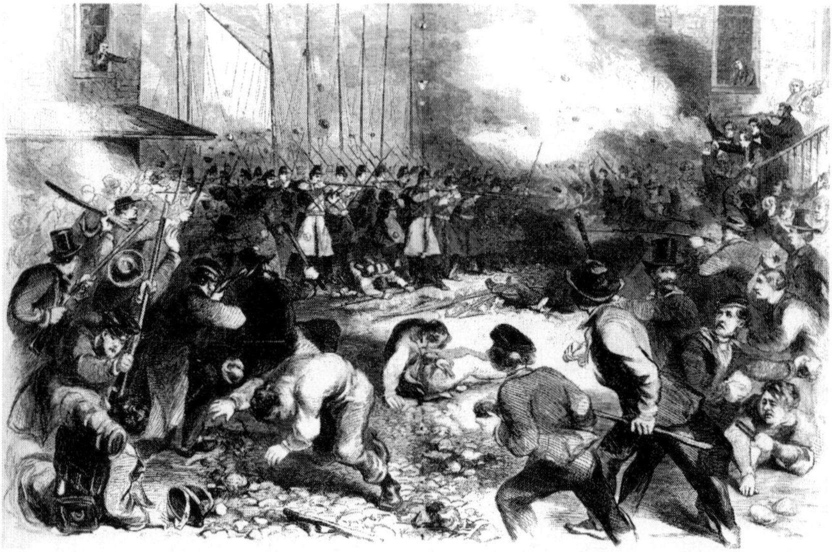

The 6th Massachusetts Militia under attack in Baltimore (*Library of Congress*)

Confederacy. In a state referendum held on May 23, 1861, Virginians voted in favor of secession, an action that threatened the safety of Washington itself. Union troops responded by crossing the Potomac River and seizing the city of Alexandria, directly opposite the capital. Colonel Elmer Ellsworth led the expedition. While he was in the act of hauling down a Confederate flag at the Marshall House Hotel, the owner struck him down, making the twenty-four-year-old colonel the war's first martyr. President Lincoln held a funeral service for Ellsworth in the East Room of the White House, after which the victim's lifeless body was carried down Pennsylvania Avenue to the Capitol. Line after line of soldiers led the procession, their arms reversed, their drums muffled, their flags furled. Four white horses pulled the coffin, which was draped with an American flag. Ellsworth's own troops trailed after the coffin, their heads bowed in grief, followed by a riderless horse, symbolizing its owner's fall, and the torn and bloody flag of secession that Ellsworth had died trying to lower. Bringing up the rear were the president and his cabinet, common mourners with the throng. Barton watched the cortege from the Treasury Building. She considered it "one of the most imposing and touching sights I ever witnessed or perhaps ever shall. . . . Not one inch of earth or space could I see," she recalled, "only one dense living, swaying, moving mass of humanity."[18]

Meanwhile, fresh volunteers by the thousands crowded into Washington, intent on protecting the capital and crushing the rebellion. The War Department organized the new troops into the Army of Northeastern Virginia and placed them under the command of Brig. Gen. Irvin McDowell. Pressured by the Lincoln administration to take action, the inexperienced general crossed the Potomac River into Virginia and engaged Confederate forces in battle along Bull Run, a sluggish creek located near the town of Manassas, twenty-five miles southwest of the capital. McDowell initially gained the upper hand, but the rebels rallied and by the end of the day swept the Union Army from the field. By nightfall, the battle was over.

For days wounded Union soldiers by the hundreds trickled back into the capital.[19] The army's medical department was unprepared for the conflict, and there were few hospitals available. To handle the influx of wounded men, it transformed public buildings into makeshift infirmaries. Barton witnessed the soldiers' suffering first hand. She frequently visited Massachusetts men confined to the hospitals and in one case purchased a cemetery plot for a deceased soldier in the city's Congressional Burying Ground.[20]

Barton was then in her thirty-ninth year. An acquaintance described her as being "of about medium height, a brunette in complexion, with dark but expressive eyes, and a form and figure which, though well rounded indicate great powers of endurance. She is not technically beautiful," he admitted, "but her features have much expression, and she possesses, unconsciously, that magnetic power which attracts others to her, and makes them ready to do her bidding."[21] Barton had never married and had no children of her own, and as time went on she came to view the army as her family and its young soldiers as sons or younger brothers. No longer was she the timid, diffident child who feared giving offense. With age had come self-confidence. She was not afraid to stand up for herself or for others, particularly the sick and wounded men under her care. She took delight in helping them and in receiving their love and gratitude in return.

As the war entered its second year, stories reached Barton about suffering within the army itself. Although the medical department had created general hospitals in cities such as Washington and Alexandria, care for sick and wounded soldiers at the front remained woefully deficient. Barton longed to assist soldiers there but feared that the men might treat her with disrespect. She later wrote, "I was strong, and thought I ought to go to the rescue of the men who fell. But I struggled long and hard with my sense of propriety, with the appalling fact that I was a woman, whispering in one ear, and the groans of suffering men . . . thundering in the other."[22] Her father vanquished those doubts. Stephen Barton had been a soldier himself. In the spring of 1862, at the age of eighty-seven, his health failed him and he stopped eating. Notified by relatives that the end was near, Clara rushed to his side. While there, she explained her dilemma to him. In reply, he assured her that if she acted like a lady the soldiers would treat her like one.[23]

Stephen's assurances gave Clara the courage she needed to pursue her goal. While he was yet alive, she shot off a letter to Governor Andrew Curtin of Massachusetts asking for permission to go to Roanoke Island, on the North Carolina coast, to "administer comfort to our brave men . . . and do with my might, whatever my hands find to do."[24] She offered to serve without pay. She chose Roanoke because the 21st Massachusetts was there. The regiment had been organized in Worcester, and it included many friends and former students. A woman of strong loyalties, Barton believed her first duty was to them. Governor Curtin referred her request to the surgeon in charge at Roanoke, who denied it without comment. "He probably thought I shall prove a fussy unreasonable, or meddlesome lady requiring more waiting upon than I did for others," she reflected, "or weakly, and should grow faint hearted at the first discouragement and get sick or home sick, or possibly self conceited and set up an opposition to the surgical regulators, a hundred things he was justified in suspecting as he knew nothing of me, and of course the safe way was to keep me at home. Under the circumstances he was wise," she concluded. In the future, she would not be so philosophical.[25]

Stephen Barton died on March 21, 1862, having gone for more than thirty days without food. He died at 10:16 in the evening, holding his daughter's hand.[26] Following his funeral, Clara returned to Washington and resumed her work at the Patent Office. By then spring had arrived, and with it came a resumption of hostilities. In April, Maj. Gen. George B. McClellan, the Army of the Potomac's new commander, took his army down the Chesapeake Bay to Fort Monroe, Virginia, at the mouth of the James River. Using the fort as his base, he slowly began working his way toward Richmond, defeating the Confederates at Yorktown and Williamsburg before General Robert E. Lee finally beat him back in a series of battles just outside the Southern capital itself. The Peninsula Campaign, as it came to be known, resulted in more than 20,000 Union casualties.

Hospital ships brought the sick and wounded back to Washington. Barton and others met the ships at the wharves with bandages and stimulants, doing whatever they could to alleviate the soldiers' suffering. It was useful work, but Barton still felt like she should be doing more. She knew the real need was at the front or, as she termed it, "between the bullet and the hospital." To go there, however, required permission from the authorities. "I should go in *five* minutes if I could be told that I might," she wrote her cousin Leander Poor, himself a soldier in the army. "I know I should do my work faithfully, and dont think I should either run, or complain if I were left under fire." She would soon have a chance to test that prediction.[27]

FREDERICKSBURG, AUGUST 1862

Having defeated McClellan and temporarily secured the safety of Richmond, Gen. Robert E. Lee marched north. His goal was to defeat Maj. Gen. John Pope's Army of Virginia in the northern part of the state before McClellan could come to his aid. Fredericksburg was the linchpin connecting the two federal armies. Standing at the fall line of the Rappahannock River, about halfway between Richmond and Washington, the picturesque old town was a regional transportation center. From it, roads radiated north, south, east, and west into the surrounding countryside. Of even greater importance, the Richmond, Fredericksburg, and Potomac Railroad passed

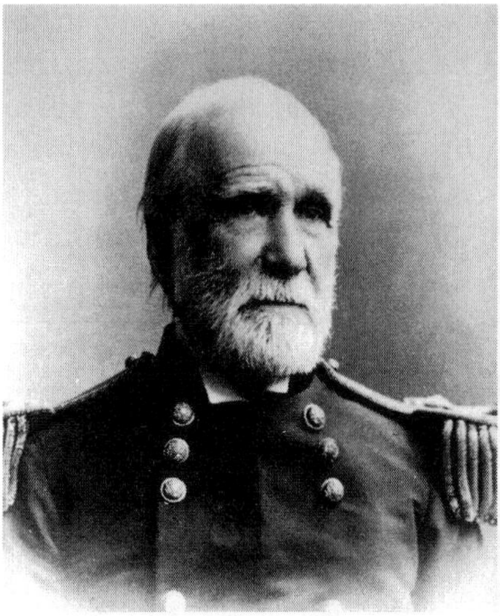
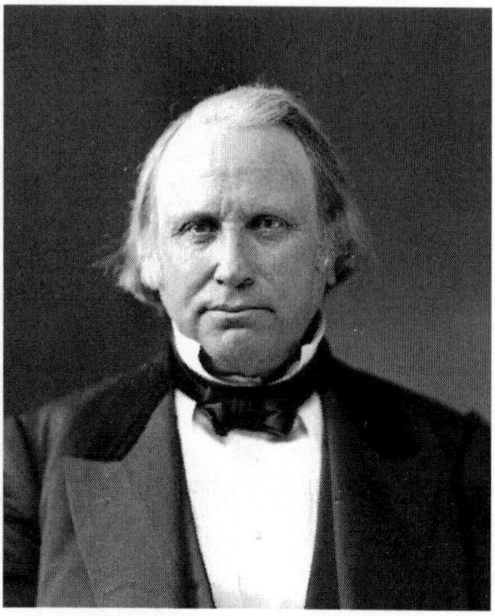

General Daniel H. Rucker, left (*United States Quartermaster Museum, Fort Lee, Virginia*); Senator Henry Wilson, right. (*Library of Congress*)

through the town on its way from Aquia Landing on the Potomac River to Richmond, providing a useful artery of supply to Union armies marching on the Confederate capital. Rebel forces had occupied Fredericksburg early in the war, but by the summer of 1862 Brig. Gen. Rufus King's Union division held the town, providing a tenuous connection between McClellan and Pope. It was here that Clara Barton would begin her work among the armies.

Barton probably chose Fredericksburg for the same reason she chose Roanoke Island: the 21st Massachusetts was there. Following Lee's victory over McClellan on the Peninsula, the War Department had ordered Maj. Gen. Ambrose E. Burnside and his Ninth Corps from North Carolina to Fredericksburg to reinforce McClellan and Pope in crushing Lee. With Burnside came twelve regiments, including the 21st Massachusetts. How Barton learned that the 21st was on its way to Fredericksburg is unknown, but there are two likely sources: Senator Henry Wilson and Col. (later Brig. Gen.) Daniel H. Rucker. Wilson was chairman of the Senate Committee on Military Affairs and one of the most powerful men in Washington. He had met Barton in the spring of 1861 and was instantly beguiled by her. "I called on him one day at the Capitol," she told a friend, "and he called on me every day after as long as he staid, so we got to be quite good friends." The senator took an unusual interest in the Massachusetts native, offering to help her overcome any problems she might encounter while in the city. As the war progressed, he would repeatedly use his influence to assist her in cutting through governmental red tape.[28] Rucker was chief quartermaster of the army's Washington Depot, a position that gave him control over millions of dollars' worth of military equipment. Apparently, he too fell under Barton's spell. During the war he kept her abreast of military developments and liberally provided her with wagons, teamsters, and commissary stores for her enterprises. Nothing that was in Rucker's power to give was denied to her. Without his and Wilson's assistance, Barton never could have achieved her goals.[29] As she later told a cousin, the two men were "*very good friends* to have if one is in the army."[30]

Before Barton could leave for Fredericksburg, she had to attend to several matters. First, she had to get a leave of absence from her job at the Patent Office. Leaving her job, even for a short time, posed a problem, for Barton relied on her salary to pay the rent on her Washington apartment. Fortunately, a male colleague stepped forward and offered to assume her duties and split his wages with her.[31] Next, she had to secure a pass to the front. According to Linus Brockett, she did this through Richard H. Coolidge, a medical inspector in the army.[32] How Barton became acquainted with Coolidge is unknown, but she probably crossed paths with him during his rounds of the Washington hospitals. Last, she needed to find someone to accompany her to the front. Barton was extremely sensitive about her reputation. Despite her father's assurances, she feared she might expose herself to scandal and malicious gossip if she visited the army alone. It simply was not done. To safeguard her honor, she felt it necessary to have a male escort or, better still, to attach herself to a group.

Fortunately, Anna Carver, Archibald G. Shaver, and Cornelius M. Welles agreed to go with her.[33] Carver was a middle-aged, married woman from Philadelphia who worked with the Penn Relief Association, an organization created by Hicksite Quakers to assist

Union soldiers.[34] Shaver, by contrast, was a thirty-two-year-old art instructor who hailed from New York. As a boy, he had caught his leg in a threshing machine, an accident that had left him lame. He had moved to Washington early in the war and, like Barton, made himself useful by bringing food to the troops "and rendering such aid as he could." He probably met her while engaged in those activities. In appearance, Shaver described himself as "Five feet 5 inches English measure, Forehead Medium h[e]ight, Eyes dark blue, Nose crooked, Mouth small, Chin narrow, Hair Auburn, with Moustache, and slight whisker on chin, Complexion light. Face Oval, & rather thin." In 1864, he would become general superintendent of the Second Army Corps hospitals, a demanding job that ruined his health. He died two years later, and as his obituary noted, as much a casualty of the war "as if he had died on the field of battle."[35]

Thirty-four-year-old Cornelius Welles had led the most interesting life of Barton's three companions. As a young man, he had become a Christian and dedicated his life to God. He initially worked among the poor in Hartford, Connecticut, but later went to California and Australia as a missionary. In 1855, he returned to Hartford to open a Mission Sunday School. For two years, he labored among the outcasts of the city: its poor, its prostitutes, its alcoholics, and its prisoners. Then he was off again, this time to Brazil and England. In 1859, Welles returned to the United States, opening a mission in New York City. In 1862, he sailed to Port Royal, South Carolina, to educate the newly freed bondsmen of that region. He remained there for just a few months, however, before going to Washington at the request of the Free Mission Society to establish a system of schools for freed slaves and their children. There he met Barton and agreed to accompany her on her trip to the army.[36]

Barton and her companions departed Washington on August 2, 1862, taking with them four boxes of supplies and two trunks. The trip got off to a rough start. Upon reaching the wharf they discovered their ship had committed an infraction and been compelled to leave the pier. Undaunted, Barton went to see Col. Rucker, who arranged for her party to take passage on a tugboat departing later in the day. The ship sailed down the Potomac and turned right into Aquia Creek, docking at the Union supply base at Aquia Landing, Virginia.

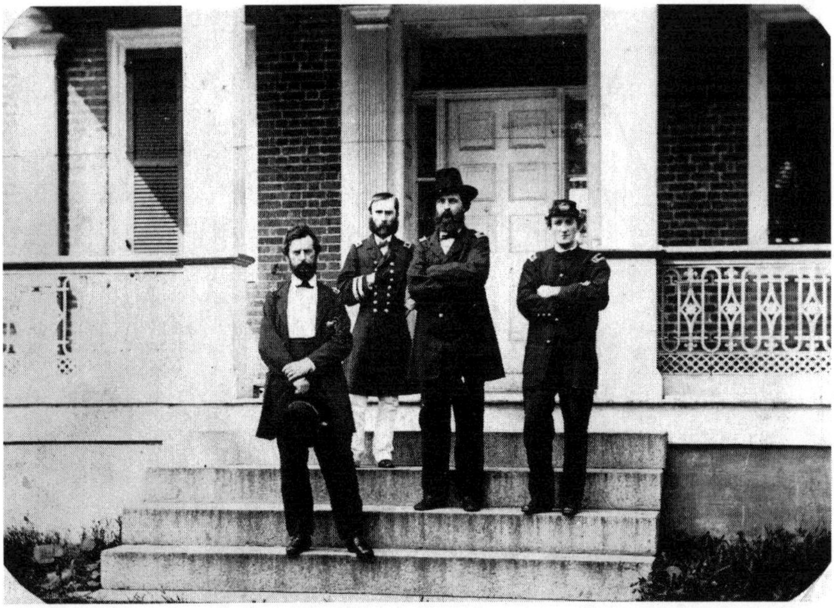

Rufus King (left) and his staff at the Lacy House (*Wisconsin Historical Society*)

Barton and her friends remained there overnight before taking a train to Fredericksburg on August 3.[37] They immediately proceeded to General King's headquarters at the Lacy House, across the Rappahannock River from Fredericksburg. Also known as Chatham, the eighteenth-century structure was the property of Maj. James Horace Lacy, an officer in the Confederate army. In coming months, Barton would come to know the building and its grounds well.[38]

On August 4, Barton crossed the Rappahannock and visited the men of the 21st New York, a regiment in King's command. She then made her way to a woolen mill at the northern end of town that Union forces had converted into a military hospital. While there, she witnessed the first of many amputations she would see over the next three years.[39] The 21st Massachusetts arrived on the same day as Barton. She called upon the regiment the next day, meeting with its commander, Col. William S. Clark, and its surgeon, Calvin Cutter. The three instantly hit it off. From that day on, Barton considered the 21st her "pet regiment," while its soldiers, for their part, referred to her as their "sister of mercy."[40]

Barton's sojourn in Fredericksburg lasted just two days. After meeting with Clark and Cutter she returned to Washington to bring up supplies for the 8th and 11th Connecticut, two other regiments in Burnside's corps. At least, that was her intention. While she was in the capital, however, news arrived that Lee had attacked Pope's army at Cedar Mountain, an isolated prominence a few miles south of Culpeper Court House, Virginia. Delegating to Welles responsibility for delivering the supplies to Fredericksburg, Barton set off at once for the scene of conflict. For the first time in her life she would be entering an active war zone.[41]

CULPEPER COURT HOUSE

Barton departed for the front on August 13, four days after the Battle of Cedar Mountain. With her went Anna Carver, Archibald Shaver, and Gardner Tufts, head of the Massachusetts state relief agency in Washington.[42] Taking the Orange and Alexandria Railroad, the party rumbled southwest over sixty miles of track to the town of Culpeper Court House, where Union surgeons had established their hospitals after the battle. It was a scene far worse than Barton had witnessed either in Washington or in Fredericksburg. "The floors of houses were covered with the wounded," wrote Tufts, "lying on the bare planks in blood and filth, with but little clothing, and in some cases perfectly naked. Some with legs shot off; others with arms off; and others wounded in different parts of the body."[43]

Sanitation was a top priority. With the help of others, Barton and her friends proceeded to clean one of the wards. They moved all the wounded soldiers to one side of the room while they scrubbed the other. They then reversed the process until the entire room was clean. Once that was done, they distributed new clothing and sheets among the soldiers and did everything in their power to make them comfortable. Union and Confederate soldiers alike shared the room. The Southern soldiers assumed that Barton was a local woman and asked her for clothing and sheets too. Their faces fell when they learned that she was from Massachusetts, supposing they would get no favors from someone who came from such a hotbed of abolitionism. But to their surprise Barton returned with the very items they sought and exhibited the same kindness toward them as she did toward the men in blue.[44]

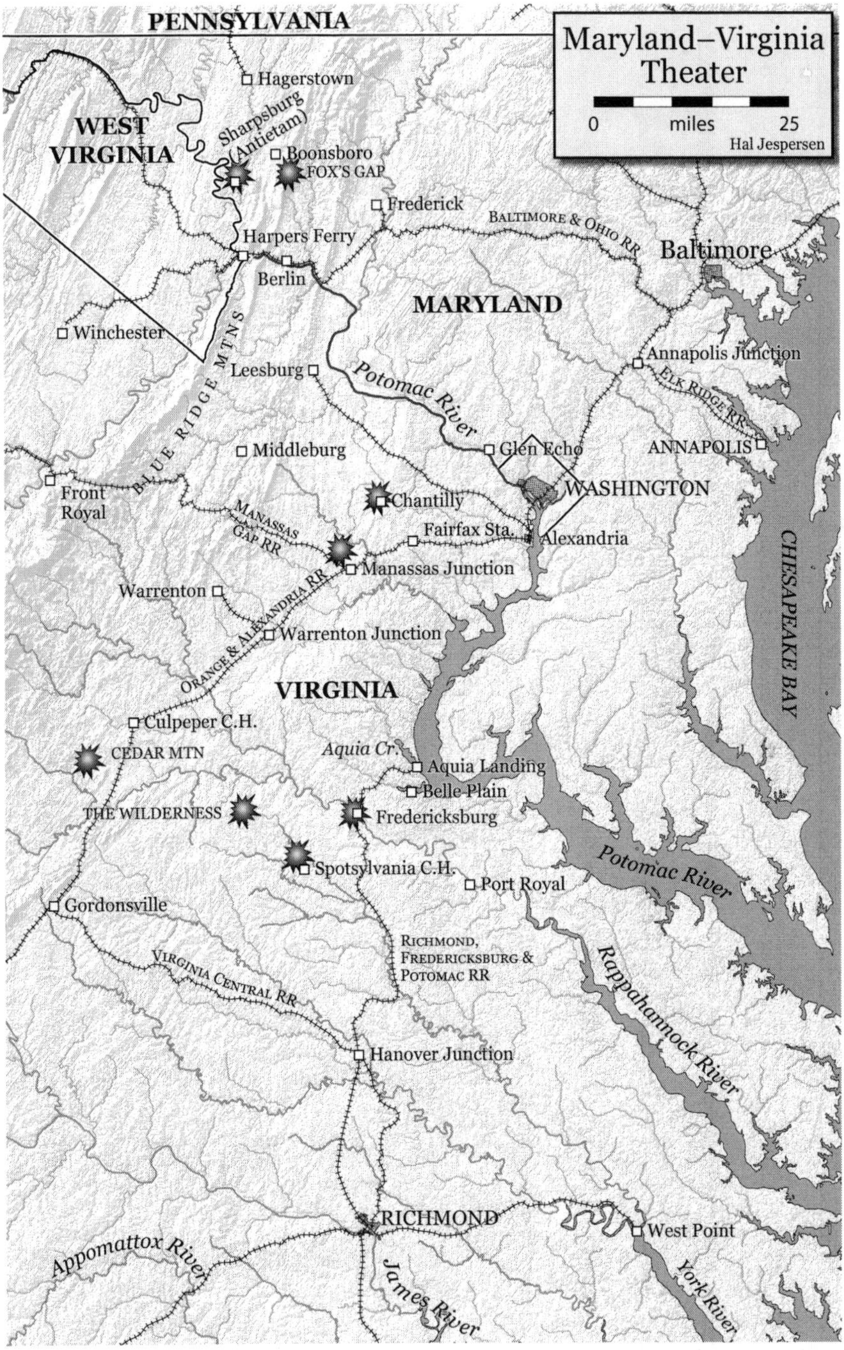
Maryland–Virginia Theater
0 miles 25
Hal Jespersen
PENNSYLVANIA
WEST VIRGINIA
MARYLAND
VIRGINIA
Hagerstown
Sharpsburg (Antietam)
Boonsboro
FOX'S GAP
Frederick
BALTIMORE & OHIO RR
Baltimore
Harpers Ferry
Berlin
Winchester
BLUE RIDGE MTNS
Leesburg
Potomac River
Annapolis Junction
ELK RIDGE RR
ANNAPOLIS
Glen Echo
WASHINGTON
Middleburg
Front Royal
Chantilly
MANASSAS GAP RR
Fairfax Sta.
Alexandria
Manassas Junction
Warrenton
ORANGE & ALEXANDRIA RR
Warrenton Junction
CHESAPEAKE BAY
Culpeper C.H.
CEDAR MTN
Aquia Cr.
Aquia Landing
Belle Plain
THE WILDERNESS
Fredericksburg
Spotsylvania C.H.
Port Royal
Potomac River
Gordonsville
RICHMOND, FREDERICKSBURG & POTOMAC RR
VIRGINIA CENTRAL RR
Rappahannock River
Hanover Junction
RICHMOND
West Point
Appomattox River
James River
York River

Major James L. Dunn wrote an account of Barton at Culpeper. Dunn was a surgeon in Pope's army, serving at the front.[45] In a letter written ten weeks later, he claimed that Barton appeared at his hospital at midnight bringing much-needed supplies. "She supplied us with everything"; he wrote, "and while the shells were bursting in every direction, took her course to the hospital on our right, where she found everything wanting again. After doing everything she could on the field, she returned to Culpepper." Unfortunately, Dunn's account of Barton's providential arrival disagrees with the New Englander's own diary. According to Barton, she did not reach the front until August 13, long after the cannon fell silent. Her diary says nothing about her visiting the front; on the contrary, it indicates that she stayed at Culpeper's Seminary Hospital the day she arrived and that she later proceeded to the Main Street Hospital, where she "found much suffering."[46] The diary likewise belies Barton's own claim made in later years that she labored in Culpeper "for five days without sleep or food (worthy of the name)" and that she "barely escaped capture" by the Confederates. It indicates clearly that she returned to Washington after just two days and never came close to an armed rebel.[47]

Before leaving Culpeper, Barton scribbled off a letter to a "Dear Old-Time Friend" that she may have intended for publication. Significantly, it says nothing about her visiting the battlefield or escaping capture, but it does provide a vivid description of a Culpeper hospital.

> Not among the din and carnage of battle, the whizzing of bullets, and thunder of guns, but here, in the dreary midnight, among the painfully moving forms, scarce visible by the glimmering light, which shoots fitfully across some knitted brow or compressed lip, just serving to show from which victim the last half smothered sigh escaped, as if it were unmanly to confess even so much of suffering—here, without a single convenience of life, without one cheering thought or view—my mind wanders out to you amid all the comforts of your invalid chamber at home, and you will pardon the disagreeable intrusions of my broken pencilings.
>
> I said we had no conveniences. We have one article of furniture—A BROAD TABLE!—and the DEATH I have seen upon it

> to-day. Oh, God! how precious! From the golden ringlets of the fair cheeked boy, the weeping, waiting, mother's idol, to the blood matted and tangled locks of the sterner, braver man, who has faced death on many a field, stretched like the broad trunk of some noble tree, to be shorn of its lightning riven branches. The bright stream that t[r]ickles from the edges to the floor—is it wine? Ah, who shall count the value of the wine of life?

Barton explained that she and her companions had rushed to the scene of action as soon as they had reliable information that a battle had taken place. "From that hour there has come to neither of us a moment's rest; want and suffering lay on every side, our ample stores diminished with a rapidity truly appalling when we looked upon so many brave and noble patriots needing everything—possessing nothing. . . . But I gaze upon these men through blinding tears of admiration and respect, and sing in my heart, 'It is well to be a soldier.'"[48] The last sentence refers to Barton herself. As a little girl, she had eagerly imbibed stories of her father's military exploits and had longed to be a soldier herself. Now she was living out that fantasy. Although she had been at the front for just a matter of days, already she had come to identify herself with those she served. In her mind, she was not merely helping the soldiers, she was one of them.

FAIRFAX STATION

After his victory at Cedar Mountain, Lee advanced toward Washington, drubbing John Pope's Army of Virginia twenty-five miles outside the city on the rolling fields of Manassas, the same ground on which the first battle of the war had been fought. Twenty thousand men fell in three days of brutal combat there. Many of the Union soldiers wounded in that battle made their way to Fairfax Station, seeking trains that would carry them to hospitals in the rear.

Barton was back in Washington when news of the battle arrived, having returned from Culpeper Court House on August 15. At once she made preparations to return to the front. With her went her friend Cornie Welles and at least four other people, including fifty-two-year-old Almira Fales. A New York native, Fales was mother to no fewer than four children and eight stepchildren. Although the war was little more than a year old, she already had considerable

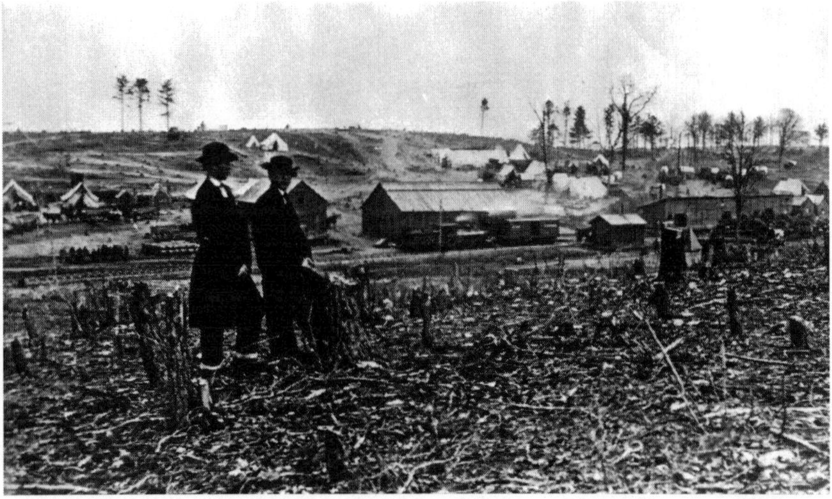

Fairfax Station, Virginia. (*Library of Congress*)

experience as a nurse, having served with Union armies at Shiloh, Tennessee; Corinth, Mississippi; and on the Virginia Peninsula.[49] As Barton left her apartment and headed for the front, she dashed off a hasty note to her brother David saying that if anything happened to her he should come and get her effects. Clearly, she anticipated danger.[50]

Barton and her party rode west on the Orange and Alexandria Railroad for fifteen miles to Fairfax Station. They arrived at 10 A.M., August 31, amid a steady rain. As they stepped onto the platform, a shocking sight met their eyes. Crowded around the station were hundreds—perhaps thousands—of wounded soldiers, their mangled forms carpeting the hill slope between the depot and nearby St. Mary's Church. Fairfax Station was a hospital in name only. It had little organization, few supplies, and no shelter. Even food was in short supply. To the small quantity of hard crackers and coffee provided by the army, Barton and her colleagues contributed food items sent to them by women in the North. Still it was not enough. As the hours wore on and supplies ran low, she recalled that they "took the meat from our own sandwiches & gave it to [the soldiers], and broke the bread into wine & water to feed the poor sinking wretches as they lay in the ambulances."[51]

Barton had brought just two water buckets, five tin cups, three plates, one camp kettle, one stew pan, and a two-quart tin dish to prepare and distribute the food—far too little for the task at hand. "O how I needed stores on that field," she lamented.[52] Fortunately, among her supplies were several large crates crammed with fruits and preserves. She not only put the food to use but the containers too. "Every can, jar, bucket, bowl, cup, or tumbler, when emptied, that instant became a vehicle of mercy to convey some preparation of mingled bread and wine or soup or coffee to some helpless, famishing sufferer," she recalled. By scrimping and innovating, she was able to feed all the soldiers she encountered. The experience taught her a valuable lesson: in the future, she would bring more supplies.[53]

Lanterns also were in short supply that week, and as night fell over the region, workers risked treading on the wounded soldiers lying at their feet. Candles alleviated the problem, but they introduced an even greater danger: fire. In lieu of bedding, surgeons had scattered hay across the ground, and despite the rain the "slightest accident, the mere dropping of a light, would have enveloped in flames this whole mass of helpless men," Barton recalled.[54] Throughout the night she and other workers moved gingerly among the wounded "in terror lest someones candle fall *into the hay* and consume them all."[55]

Barton spent three hours that night caring for a single soldier, Pvt. Hugh Johnson of the 104th New York. The twenty-two-year-old Irish immigrant had been shot through the stomach and was not expected to live. In his delirium, he initially imagined Barton to be his sister, an illusion she chose not to dispel. Johnson drifted off to sleep after just ten minutes, but Barton remained at his side until morning. By then, he had regained his senses. With difficulty, he told her that he was an only son and that, when he died, his mother would want to retrieve his body. Even though he knew that the trip might kill him, he insisted on being sent back to Washington. Barton gratified the young man's wishes and sent him back on the next train. On September 5, after returning to Washington, she visited Armory Square Hospital to check on Johnson, but she was too late. He had died the previous night. Before she left the hospital, a chaplain

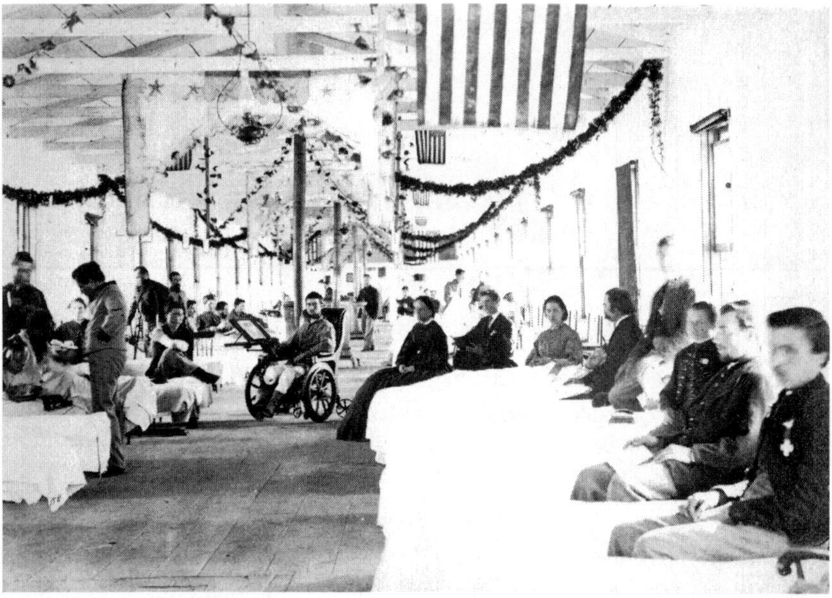

Armory Square Hospital. (*Library of Congress*)

directed her attention to a nearby wagon onto which soldiers had loaded the young man's coffin. Beside the vehicle stood two grieving women: Johnson's mother and his sister, Mary. Because of Barton, they had been at the young man's side when he died and were able to take his body home and give it a proper burial.[56] Barton left the hospital without speaking to the women, wishing, she said, to "be spared the scene and the thanks." She did hear from them later, however. Her friend John J. Elwell later claimed to have seen "a tear covered letter from the boy's New England mother, thanking Clara Barton for giving her the privilege of being with her dying son and of burying him with his kindred."[57]

It is a touching story but unfortunately it does not square with the facts. Records show that Johnson was shot on August 30 and died in Washington two days later, on Monday, September 1, far too soon for Johnson's mother and sister to have joined him there from New York. By Barton's own admission, they did not reach Armory Square Hospital until September 3, two days after he died. Having the women arrive prior to Johnson's death added poignancy to the story, however, and validated Barton's judgment in sending him to the rear, even though the jarring train ride may in fact have contributed to his death.[58]

Wounded soldiers continued to arrive at Fairfax Station by the thousands for twenty-four hours after Johnson's departure. At least seven of them Barton recognized as former pupils. She later recalled "the shock and heart-breaking sensation of finding myself suddenly in the presence of a mutilated, perishing human form" whom she had known and loved in more innocent times. One of these was Charley Hamilton, a fair-haired young man who had come to the hospital with a butchered right arm. At first, Barton did not recognize him. However, he recognized her instantly, and when she leaned over to cover him, he grabbed her around the neck with his good arm and began sobbing. "And you do not know me?" he asked. "I am Charley Hamilton, who used to carry your satchel home from school." Barton looked closely at him and saw in Hamilton's "wan, distorted features, the bright happy face" that had once looked to her "for counsel and approval." In his blood-matted hair she saw the "fair locks" that had "tossed in the wind as he played," and in the "dead, cold hand hanging at his side" awaiting the surgeon's saw, she recognized "the little boyish fingers" that she had once "taught to trace his name." To Barton, it was like looking at one of her own children. She would have stayed with him, but others needed her care now, many of them more badly injured than Charley. Barton tried to make her former pupil comfortable and perhaps offered words of encouragement, but in her heart she knew the wound would leave him permanently disabled, if indeed it did not kill him. "Poor Charley," she thought to herself as she hurried away, "that mangled arm will never carry a satchel again."[59]

Barton and her colleagues kept busy throughout the day feeding the new arrivals, drawing water for them, and dressing their wounds. Fortunately, they had help. Nearby were fifty Union soldiers who had been arrested for various infractions, whom the provost marshal placed at the hospital's disposal. For the tired and overworked aid workers, the prisoners were a godsend. They "dug graves and gathered and buried the dead, bore mangled men over the rough ground in their arms, loaded cars, built fires, made soup, and administered it," Barton recalled.[60] Perhaps the most valuable task performed by the prisoners was lifting the wounded soldiers onto the trains. "We sent up the train with 1250, next 1000, next 1100, next 940, and so on," Barton wrote Archibald Shaver and others after returning to Washington. "Still the ambulances came down and the cars went out and we worked on."[61] Many of those being evacuated had been on the field for two or three days and were literally dying for lack of nourishment. At Barton's suggestion, the surgeons ordered that every wounded soldier be examined and fed before being taken from the wagons and placed aboard the trains. She remembered doing much of this work herself, "climbing from the wheel to the brake of every wagon, speaking to and feeding with my own hands each soldier until he expressed himself satisfied."[62] That was a gross exaggeration, of course. For Barton to have personally fed each of the thousands of soldiers who passed through Fairfax Station, as she averred, would have been impossible.

Among those at Fairfax Station on September 1 was James Dunn, the surgeon who had met Barton at Culpeper three weeks earlier. Dunn later wrote a letter praising Barton's actions at Fairfax Station, but, like his account of Barton's actions at Culpeper, it is riddled with errors. For instance, he claimed that Barton initially delivered supplies to his field hospital at Manassas on August 29 "while the battle was raging its fiercest." She reached the battlefield, he wrote, "with her mules almost dead, having made forced marches from Washington to the army." However, a letter written by Barton at the time clearly states that she did not reach the front until August 31 and that she traveled by train, not by wagon. Moreover, she never got within ten miles of the Manassas battlefield. Dunn went on to say that he encountered Barton again at Fairfax Station on September 1, when his benefactress appeared on an incoming train "to again supply us with bandages, brandy, wine, prepared soup, jellies, meal, and every article that could be thought of." However, Barton had been at Fairfax Station for a full day when Dunn arrived, and by then she had exhausted her limited stores. Such fundamental mistakes wholly discredit Dunn's testimony.[63]

Lee trounced Pope in two days of heavy fighting at Manassas, forcing him to withdraw to Washington. Not content with merely defeating his enemy, Lee dispatched Maj. Gen. "Stonewall" Jackson on a march around Pope's right flank in an effort to intercept the Union army in its retreat and destroy it. The two forces collided on September 1 near the village of Chantilly, grappling with one another amid the thunder and lightning of a summer storm. Although the battle took place fully eight miles from Fairfax Station, to Barton it seemed much closer, "about *two* miles distant." She interpreted the battle not as an attempt by Lee to destroy Pope's army but rather as an effort by him to capture the Union field hospital at Fairfax Station. Only stiff fighting by the 21st Massachusetts, she believed, thwarted the effort. "We sat down in our tent and waited to see them break in upon us," she wrote, but the Ninth Corps held the Confederates back. "The *old 21st Mass* lay between us & the enemy & they *couldn't pass,*" she declared. The prospect of being captured unnerved Almira Fales. As the fighting raged in the distance, she insisted on returning to Washington for additional supplies. She suggested that Barton join her, but the younger woman adamantly refused to leave her post. With an air of self-righteousness, Barton later told audiences that she "begged to be excused from accompanying her [Fales] as the ambulances were up to the field for more and I knew *I* should *never leave a wounded man there* if I knew it, though I were taken prisoner 40 times." Fales departed alone.[64]

During the night Pope broke contact with the Confederate army and hurried east, seeking refuge behind the capital's defenses. The medical department joined the retreat on September 2. "We knew this was the last," Barton wrote her friends. "We put the thousand wounded we had then into the train[.] I took one car load of them Mrs M[orrell] another. the men took to horse. we steamed off and two hours after there was *no Fairfax Station*[.]"[65] In later years, Barton heightened the drama of the situation by turning the retreat into a hairbreadth escape. She told listeners that an officer personally came to her that afternoon with a warning that Confederate horsemen were approaching. But like before, Barton refused to leave the depot until every wounded man had been safely evacuated. An hour later, the same officer returned to report that the enemy forces were only a short distance away. "Now is your time," Barton recalled him saying. "The cavalry is already breaking over the hills. Try the train. It will go through unless they have flanked and cut the bridge a mile above us. In that case, I have a reserve horse for you, and you must take your chances of escape across the country." In two minutes, she wrote, "I was on the train. The last wounded man at the station was also on. The conductor stood with a torch, which he applied to a pile of combustible material beside the track, and as we rounded the curve which took us from view, we saw the station ablaze and a troop of Rebel Cavalry dashing down the hill."[66] It was a thrilling story, but it probably never happened.

The train reached Alexandria at 10 o'clock that night. Despite the lateness of the hour, loyal citizens met the locomotive at the station, bringing food for the wounded passengers. Barton helped feed the hungry men and then dined herself. It was well past midnight before she crossed the Potomac River and found rest in her Washington apartment. During the three days she had been gone, she had slept little more than an hour—or so she claimed. Nevertheless, she was ready to set off again at a moment's notice. As she told her friends, "I am well & strong and wait to go again if I have need." That time would come sooner than she imagined.[67]

2

Antietam

"THE SHADOW OF DEATH"

Following his victory at Second Manassas, General Robert E. Lee led his army across the Potomac River into Maryland, pursued by George McClellan and the Army of the Potomac. On September 17, 1862, McClellan brought Lee to bay on the banks of Antietam Creek, where the two engaged one another in what would be America's single bloodiest day of battle. This time Clara Barton would be present at the outset of the fighting. Her earlier experiences at Culpeper Court House and Fairfax Station, she later wrote, had taught her "the folly and wickedness of remaining quietly at home until reporters and journalists told us that a battle had been fought and thousands of our men lay dying on the field without food or nursing. I had determined to anticipate trouble and meet it halfway at least." In order to anticipate trouble, however, she needed inside information about the army's movements. She got it on September 13 when a messenger arrived with a note that said, "Harpers Ferry—not a moment to be lost." Although she did not identify her informant, it was almost certainly Daniel Rucker, the man she aptly referred to as her "patron saint."[1]

Barton instantly repaired to Rucker's office and requested permission to go to Harpers Ferry, a small but strategic town at the confluence of the Potomac and Shenandoah Rivers. With a look "uncommonly full of meaning," the general granted her request, offering to send her an army wagon the next morning. Barton filled the vehicle with items that experience told her might be useful to wounded soldiers. By contrast, she took so few items for her own comfort that she was able to wrap them all in a single handkerchief. Once everything was in order, she pulled away from her house on Seventh Street and turned down Pennsylvania Avenue, rattling past civilians who were on their way to church. Cornie Welles and an army teamster joined her. For the first time, she would head to the front without the company of another woman.[2]

For a full day the wagon bounced along country roads in an effort to catch up with the Army of the Potomac, which even then was clawing its way through the gaps of South Mountain. The distant roar of artillery bespoke trouble ahead. At nightfall, Barton and her companions parked in a field beside the road, made supper, and dropped off to sleep. By the time the sun rose the next morning, they were back on the road.[3] Barton soon caught up with the army and found herself "in the midst of a train of army wagons at least ten miles in length moving in solid column." With each mile the number of stragglers increased. "Weary and sick from their late exposures and hardships, the men were failing and falling by the wayside, faint, pale, and often dying," she wrote. She passed out slices of bread to those she passed, restocking her supplies at each new village she entered.[4]

When Barton's wagon reached the town of Frederick, Maryland, it angled left and began climbing South Mountain toward Fox's Gap, where fighting had occurred just twenty-four hours earlier. The medical department had collected the wounded from the battlefield, but rebel corpses still littered the roadside and adjacent fields. Barton later claimed that she and her party "found our wheels crushing the bodies of the unburied slain," but that is certainly a fabrication. By her own account, her wagon was traveling in the wake of several hundred other vehicles, any of which would have stopped to pull a corpse out of the road. Significantly, Welles never mentioned any such incident.[5]

South Mountain was the first actual battlefield that Barton had ever visited, and it left a deep impression on her. The "mingled mass of stiffened, blackened men, horses, muskets, bayonets, knapsacks, haversacks, blankets, coats, canteens, broken wheels and cannonballs" that met her gaze, she wrote, told her all too plainly "that our troops had met a foe who madly stood his ground."[6] She and her colleagues searched in vain for any wounded soldiers who remained on the field, but they found none and soon continued on their way.[7] A short distance ahead they came upon a house being used by Confederate surgeons as a field hospital. The soldiers inside lacked food. A drove of Union cattle was passing, and surgeons asked the officer in charge if they could have one of his animals to feed their starving men. While the Union officer sympathized with their plight, he felt powerless to help. According to Barton, he was accountable for each of the oxen in the herd and did not feel authorized to give one of them away. Instead, he conspired to have one of the animals get loose and had Barton drive it into the yard of the needy Confederates. "Three years later, as I stood among the 12,000 graves of Andersonville, filled with the skeletons of the martyrs of Freedom, the victims of deliberate starvation, I could not but think how ill that day's generosity had been requited," she later told her audiences.[8]

Like many of Barton's stories, this one doesn't ring true. It's unlikely that the Commissary Department kept a strict account of the animals under its charge, but assuming that it did, it hardly explains why losing an ox would make the officer in charge less responsible than giving one away to needy prisoners. But if he did want to make it appear the animal had been lost, why involve Barton? Why not simply leave it in the yard himself? In fact, why was it necessary to leave an ox at all? Barton had a wagonload of supplies. If she wished to aid the wounded Confederates, why did she not supply them from her own stocks rather than resort to subterfuge? The story simply does not make sense.

Meanwhile, up ahead, a battle was brewing near the town of Sharpsburg. Eager to reach the front but caught behind an endless procession of wagons, Barton resorted to a shrewd ploy. Stopping in the middle of the day, she and her assistants made camp and rested.

When night arrived and the rest of the army pulled off the road to sleep, they pushed forward on the now-empty roads and by dawn found themselves ten miles ahead, just in the rear of the army's artillery train. They followed the batteries throughout the day and at dark bedded down among the men of Burnside's Ninth Corps. "In all this vast assemblage I saw no other trace of womankind," Barton wrote. "I was faint but could not eat, weary but could not sleep, depressed but could not weep. So I climbed into my wagon, tied down the cover, dropped down in the little nook I had occupied so long, and prayed God with all the earnestness of my soul to stay the morrow's strife or send us victory; and for my poor self that he impart somewhat of wisdom and strength to my heart, nerve to my arm, speed to my feet, and fill my hands for the terrible duties of the coming day. And heavy and sad I waited its approach."[9]

The sullen roar of artillery at dawn, September 17, indicated all too clearly that the day of battle had arrived. Just ahead, wrote Welles, "the work of destruction and death fairly began."[10] The battle opened on the Union right. When cavalry and artillery began moving in that direction, Barton fell in behind them with her wagon. Around 9 A.M., she and her two companions halted in a cornfield located near a grove of trees later famous as the North Woods. Union artillery thundered nearby, provoking an angry reply from Southern batteries. Their shells burst overhead but did little harm.[11]

That was not the case closer to the front. There, in the cornfield of a farmer named Miller, Union soldiers were falling by the thousands. As wounded men drifted to the rear, Barton and her colleagues tore apart a nearby haystack and began preparing makeshift beds for them. "Soon," remembered Welles, "we were entirely surrounded by those whose wounds were of the most ghastly and dangerous character, legs and arms off, and all manner of gaping wounds from shell and minié balls." Among those carried to the rear were a number of wounded Confederate officers. Like their comrades at Culpeper, they were surprised to receive from Barton and her assistants the same care as Union soldiers.[12]

Near the spot where Barton had halted stood a barn. Although it was still early in the battle, hundreds of torn and mangled soldiers had already gathered there hoping to find relief. Barton knew there

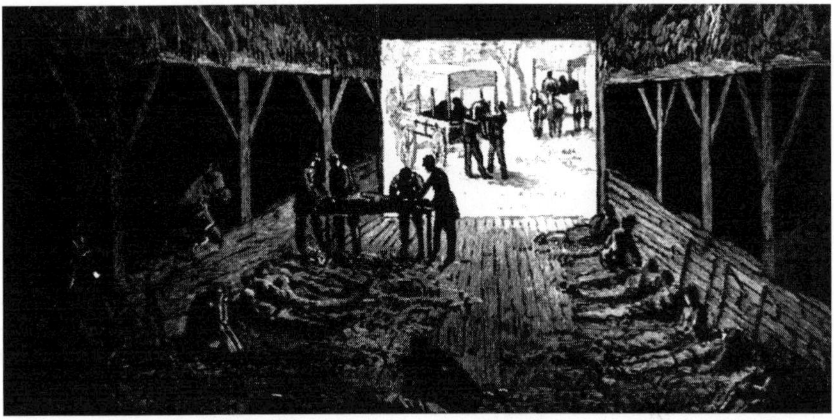

Union wounded in the Poffenberger barn. (*Library of Congress*)

must be a house nearby and that Union surgeons were probably using it as a hospital. Grabbing an armload of bandages and stimulants (probably whiskey), she followed a driveway that led through the high corn to the farmhouse of Joseph Poffenberger. Incredibly, she found herself face to face with James Dunn, the same surgeon she had encountered at both Culpeper and Fairfax Station. Medical supplies had not yet caught up with the army, and Dunn despaired of being able to treat the hundreds of men who had come to him for help. "We had expended every bandage, torn up every sheet in the house, and everything we could find," he wrote, "when who should drive up but our old friend Miss Barton, with a team loaded down with dressings of every kind, and everything we could ask for."[13]

For a moment the two faced one another, speechless. Then, as Dunn recognized Barton's features, he blurted out: "God has indeed remembered us! How did you get from Virginia here so soon and again to supply our necessities? And they are terrible. We have nothing but our instruments and the little chloroform we brought in our pockets, have torn up the last sheets we could find in this house, have not a bandage, rag, lint, or string, and all these shell-wounded men bleeding to death." The hospital was so destitute of supplies, Barton recalled, that surgeons had been compelled to dress wounds with green corn husks in lieu of bandages. Under the circumstances, her timely arrival must indeed have seemed providential.[14]

For the rest of that day and into the night Barton and Welles labored among the crowd of wounded men gathered around the Poffenberger dwelling, attempting, Welles wrote, "to stay the crimson tide where life was ebbing out, and cheer, and comfort, and restore, and nourish the poor fainting sufferers, until substantial aid could reach them, or receive the last dying message, and soothe as best we might the sudden passage through the dark valley and the shadow of death."[15] They were aided in their work by a dozen or more men who sought to escape the carnage by helping their wounded comrades to the rear. According to Linus Brockett, Barton put the shirkers to work "administering restoratives, bringing and applying water, lifting men to easier positions, stopping hemorrhages," and other useful tasks.[16]

Meanwhile, the fighting raged nearby. "The men were dragged out from under the guns and brought to us by hundreds," Barton recalled; "the smoke nearly stifled us, and the heavens turned red, and the earth shook, and the faces of the dying and dead grew ghastly bright in the lurid light of battle, and the solid shot thundered by, and the screeching shell broke over and amid, and buried themselves in the broad fields beyond us."[17] Occasionally a stray bullet or shell fragment found its mark. While Barton was bending over a wounded soldier, a bullet passed between her body and her arm. It pierced the sleeve of her dress before entering the chest of the man she was helping. He died instantly. "I have never mended that hole in my sleeve," she told later audiences. "I wonder if a soldier ever does mend a bullet hole in his coat?"[18]

At the height of the fighting, Barton encountered a man who had been shot in the face. The bullet had lodged in the bone near his right cheek. She offered to fetch a doctor, but he implored her to remove the bullet herself, apparently preferring the help of an unknown civilian to that of a trained surgeon. When Barton expressed fear that she might hurt him, the man answered: "You cannot hurt me dear lady. I can endure any pain that your hands can create. Please do it—twill relieve me so much." Barton obliged and removed the bullet. "I do not think a surgeon would have pronounced it a scientific operation," she later told audiences, "but that it was successful I dared to hope from the gratitude of the patient." How the man managed to speak so eloquently with a bullet in his jaw, she did not explain.[19]

While the members of her party "labored through that terrible day, amid the roar of the musketry and cannonading, setting broken limbs, staunching ghastly wounds, [and] bathing broken heads," Barton devoted much of her time to preparing food for the soldiers.[20] By 2 P.M., however, her helpers reported "that the last loaf of bread had been cut and the last cracker pounded." All that remained were three crates of wine. Barton ordered the men to open the containers and distribute the wine among the wounded. To their astonishment, the men discovered that the wine had been packed in Indian meal. Scrounging up some iron kettles, Barton mixed the meal with water to make gruel. Someone then suggested checking the cellar. There they discovered three barrels of flour and a bag of salt left by the Confederate army. "I shall never experience such a sensation of wealth and competency again," Barton later gushed. "From utter poverty to such riches!" As a result of the unexpected windfall, she insisted that she and her assistants not only fed the men at the Poffenberger farm but also "carried buckets of hot gruel" to wounded soldiers "for miles down the line." When she returned that night, her face was soiled by the smoke of battle and her lips and throat were parched with thirst.[21]

Darkness brought a welcome halt to the fighting, but it did not alleviate the suffering at the Poffenberger farm, where hundreds of men still awaited treatment. Many had gone inside the barn during the day to shelter themselves from exploding shells, and as night came on Barton directed her helpers to hang lanterns in and around the structure. Walking inside the house, she found the surgeon in charge staring dejectedly at the stump of a candle that was flickering on a table in front of him. In a speech delivered after the war, Barton recalled rousing the doctor from his doleful trance.

"You are tired, Doctor," she said.

He turned upon her savagely. "Tired? Yes! I am tired—tired of such heartlessness, such carelessness! Think of the condition of things. Here are at least 1000 wounded men—terribly wounded—500 of whom cannot live till daylight without attention." Motioning toward the table, he added: "That two inches of candle is all I have or can get. What can I do? How can I endure it?"

Taking the doctor by the arm, she led him to the door and pointed to the barn, now illuminated by the lanterns.

"What is that?" he asked, obviously puzzled.

"The barn is lighted," she answered, "and the house will be directly." She went on to explain that she had brought with her thirty lanterns and four boxes of candles—more than enough to get them through the night. "He looked at me a moment," she recalled, "turned away without a word, and never afterward alluded to the circumstances. But the deference which he paid me was almost painful."[22]

Surgeons worked throughout the night in an effort to treat as many wounded soldiers as possible. Barton and her comrades also kept at it. "We could not think of rest," wrote Welles, "although we had had none for two or three days; for all around us were dying men, calling for water, for friends, for God to deliver them from their miseries; some of them with the whole thigh shot off, some with both arms off some with bullets through their chest, and others with deathly wounds through which life was gradually ebbing away." Despite their best efforts, nearly half the men they were treating died by the following morning.[23] Nevertheless, Barton and Welles kept to their task throughout the night and into the next day. Only with the arrival of additional nurses and supplies after dark on September 18 could they finally enjoy the luxury of rest. Even then, the agonizing shrieks and groans of the wounded soldiers made it difficult to sleep.[24]

The Confederate army slipped away that night, leaving the Army of the Potomac in possession of the ground. Except for South Mountain, neither Barton nor Welles had ever seen a battlefield, and with the Confederates now gone they ventured forth to take a look. The ghastly sights and horrid stench sickened them, but the Confederate prisoners they met elicited only their pity. "The rebels whom we saw were, without exception, the most forlorn, wretched, hungry-looking beings we ever saw," recalled Welles. "The appearance of all, both officers and men, was uniformly ragged and dirty, many barefooted, some bare-headed, and all with *dirty shirts*. Very many of them did not hesitate to say that if they ever got freed from this *servitude*, they would never fight the North again. After spending an hour among them, we returned to our hospital."[25]

With their stock of supplies nearly gone and a new set of nurses on the scene to care for the wounded, Barton and Welles decided it was time to return to Washington. At noon, September 19, they started back, going by way of the army's left wing so that they could inquire after the welfare of friends in the Ninth Corps. On the way, recalled Welles, they stopped at no fewer than nineteen field hospitals to distribute supplies they had not used.[26] Their journey took them through the town of Boonsboro, Maryland, where Barton halted long enough to chat with the surgeon of the 124th Pennsylvania and make soup for some of the troops.[27] By then she was on her last legs. A week with little rest had made inroads on her health, and on the morning of September 20 she developed what she described as a "raging fever," experiencing great pain in her limbs. Rather than leave her at one of the many crowded hospitals in the area, her companions placed her in the bottom of their wagon and carried her the eighty-mile distance back to Washington. Barton survived the harrowing journey but remained bedridden for several days. She had a strong constitution, however, and within a week she was back on her feet, preparing for the next campaign. Her cousin Leander Poor visited her in Washington on September 29 and found her "looking just as usual," which he found remarkable considering all she had suffered. "It has been more than a common soldier could endure," he thought, "yet I find her with head, heart and hands full of business; calm, methodical and cheerful." Barton had recovered both her strength and spirit. She would need both, for even greater challenges lay ahead.[28]

3

Fredericksburg

"YOUR PLACE IS HERE"

Following the Battle of Antietam, the Army of the Potomac remained in Maryland for six weeks licking its wounds. Although the weather was ideal for military operations, Maj. Gen. George B. McClellan was unwilling to pursue the Confederates into Virginia until his army had fully recovered from its recent struggle. Even a visit by Abraham Lincoln could not make him budge. As he left McClellan to return to Washington, the frustrated president cast a backward glance at the powerful army resting in its camps. Gesturing toward the sea of tents, he asked a companion, "Do you know what this is?" When his bemused friend replied that it was the Army of the Potomac, Lincoln shook his head in weary disagreement. "So it is called, but that is a mistake; it is only McClellan's bodyguard."[1]

Toward the end of October, the Union general finally roused himself to action. On the twenty-sixth of that month, he led his army across the Potomac River back into Virginia and slowly made his way south toward the town of Warrenton. Hearing that the army was again in motion, Clara Barton hurried to Col. Rucker's office and got him to supply her with four wagons, an ambulance for her own personal use, thirty-eight mules, and a large supply of commissary stores. In addition to all of this, she appears to have had two wagons of her own. Joining her in the coming campaign were her old sidekick, Cornie Welles; a nephew, Stephen Barton; an ambulance driver with the first name of James; three teamsters named George Morton, Peter Stark, and John Mills; and a seventh man known only as Wesley, alias York.[2] The teamsters were rough sorts, unused to taking orders, and they resented Rucker placing them in a woman's charge. At first, they were uncooperative—even rebellious—but Barton claims to have won them over with kindness and insisted that by the time the men reached Fredericksburg they were devoted to her.[3]

Barton and her party left Washington and headed northwest toward the Army of the Potomac's last known location, Harpers Ferry, made famous three years earlier by John Brown. When they reached the town, however, they discovered that the army had broken camp and was crossing the Potomac River downstream at Berlin (now Brunswick), Maryland. Barton dutifully followed, but when her teamsters reached the river they refused to cross. She gave them a choice: continue forward or be dismissed. They continued forward.[4]

Mishaps attended the journey. Upon reaching the pontoon bridge, one of Peter Stark's mules broke loose, delaying the army for twenty minutes until its driver could get the animal back in its traces. Later that same day one of Barton's other men drove her largest wagon over a five-foot-tall embankment, damaging it.[5] The rest of the trip was less eventful but no less dangerous. "Our march up the Maryland hills and down the Virginia mountains was long, broken, and uncertain, harassed by the enemy both front and rear," she later told audiences. For protection, the little wagon train attached itself to Brig. Gen. Samuel Sturgis's division of the Ninth Corps, where it acted as "a general purveyor for the sick," providing food for any ailing soldiers within its reach. When the army reached Warrenton Junction, McClellan sent 1,400 infirm soldiers back to Washington. Barton and Welles accompanied them, leaving the wagons in the charge of some soldiers from the 21st Massachusetts, whom Sturgis had kindly detailed for that purpose.[6]

The night before she and Welles reached Washington, Barton sat down beside a campfire fueled by the timber of a dogwood tree. Smoke from the burning wood created an allergic reaction, causing her face to swell enormously, preventing her from seeing out of one eye. At the same time, she developed a painful inflammation in her finger, called a felon. Although she had a surgeon lance it, her hand remained sore for several days. Despite these afflictions, she returned to the front after just two weeks.[7]

In her absence the Army of the Potomac had acquired a new leader. Disappointed by McClellan's lack of aggression, President Lincoln on November 9, 1862, replaced him with Maj. Gen. Ambrose E. Burnside. In an unusual display of vigor, Burnside led the army in a hard march to Fredericksburg, thirty-five miles away. He hoped to cross the river on pontoon bridges sent from Washington and then race south toward Richmond, bringing the Confederates to battle somewhere along the way. However, his plan fell through when the bridges failed to arrive on schedule. By the time the pontoons reached Fredericksburg, in late November, Lee's army occupied the hills south and west of town, blocking his path. Temporarily checked in its southward movement, the Army of the Potomac settled into camps near Falmouth, Virginia, to await its commander's next move.

Barton and Welles rejoined the army at Falmouth in early December, bringing with them a fresh supply of hospital and general stores for the army.[8] The two traveled by ship as far as the army's supply base at Aquia Landing. There, to Barton's delight, she found an old friend on duty: Adjutant Theron E. Hall of the 21st Massachusetts. Hall had Barton's stores taken ashore and visited her on board her ship that evening. "We had a *home* chat I assure you," she later wrote to a friend.[9] That day and the next Welles distributed supplies to Union regiments camped at Aquia Landing. Meanwhile, Hall placed Barton's goods aboard a train and forwarded them to Falmouth Station, less than a mile from Fredericksburg. Barton and Welles followed. Luck was with Barton that week, for at Falmouth Station she encountered yet another acquaintance in the person of a Captain Bailey.[10] Barton explained to Bailey that she was looking for Sturgis, in whose care she had left her wagons during her absence in Washington. Bailey gave her directions to Sturgis's headquarters and promised to forward her supplies there once he could load them onto wagons.[11]

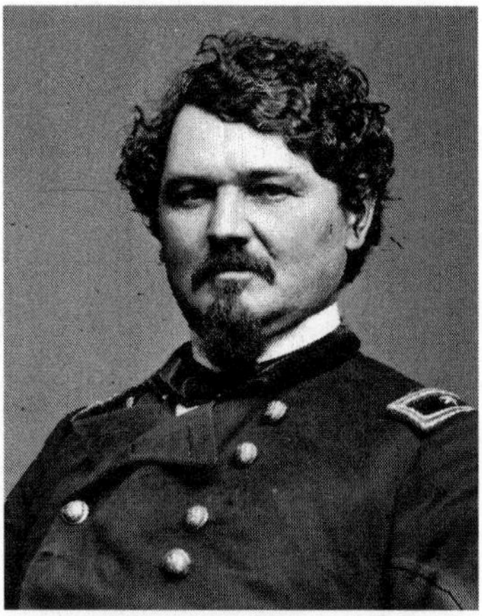

General Samuel Sturgis. (*Library of Congress*)

Sturgis commanded the Second Division of the Ninth Corps. With a round face, tousled hair, and dark goatee, he looked like a swash-buckling cavalier straight out of a Van Dyck painting. The chivalrous general greeted Barton like an honored guest. Not only did he give her use of his personal ambulance, but he also provided her with supper and arranged a "splendid serenade" on her behalf. It was the kind of attention Barton relished. "I dont know how we could have had a warmer 'welcome home' as the officers termed it," she gushed.[12]

Sturgis had his headquarters at the farmhouse of James M. S. Threshley, one and one-quarter miles east of Fredericksburg. The general arranged for Barton to lodge at the house, where she shared a room with a woman identified only as "Miss G."[13] Although Barton preferred the privacy and comfort of her own tent to a crowded building, she gratefully accepted Sturgis's offer. "My wagons are a little way from me, out of sight," she confided to a friend, "and I am wishing for a tent and stove to pitch and live near them. –the weather is cold, and the ground covered with snow, but I could make me comfortable with a good tent, floor and stove, and should prefer it to a room in a rebel house and one so generally occupied." According to Harriet Eaton, another nurse traveling with the army, Barton had four ambulances (or wagons) and seven men with her at the time.[14]

Once Barton and Welles got settled into their new quarters, they began what Welles termed "a series of visits to the regimental hospitals, supplying their wants, and administering in various ways to the comfort of these poor fellows." The weather had been cold

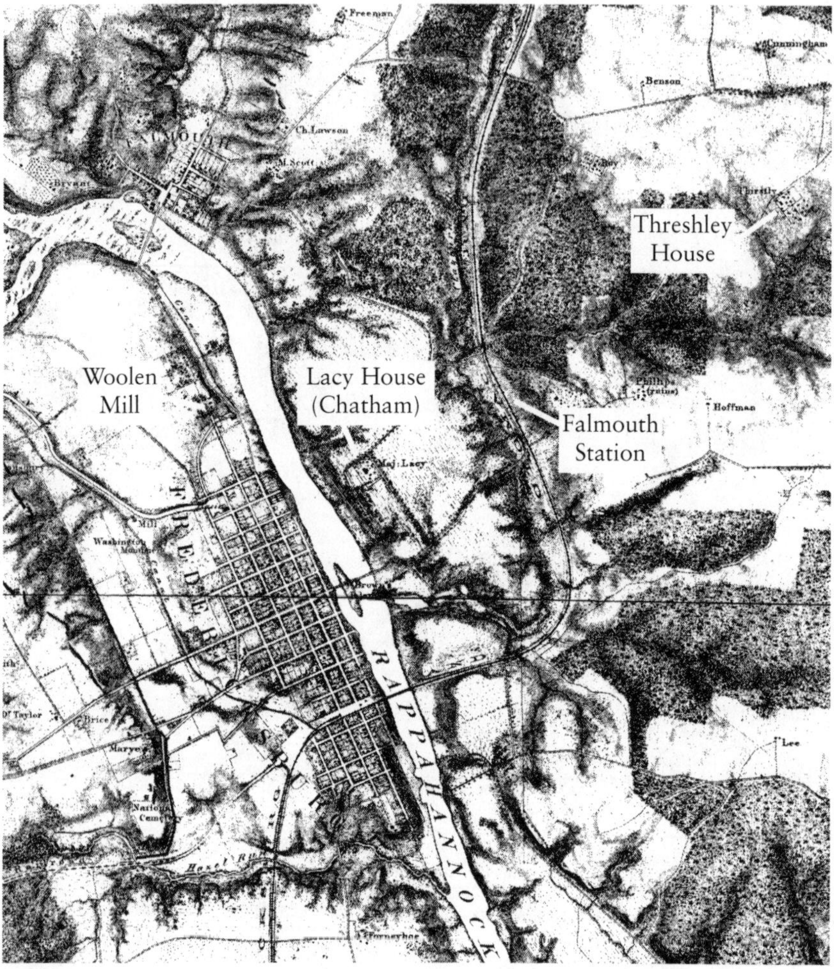

Clara Barton sites near Fredericksburg, 1862. (*Library of Congress/Author*)

and damp, and there was a great deal of sickness in the army. In one hospital alone, they found thirty-seven patients with fever. Into such settings they "brought comfort in good things, and sympathy in kind words." Doctors and patients alike welcomed their arrival. "Our soldiers appreciate the kindness of those who thus remember them, and many blessings are given to those who at home think of the soldier," wrote Welles.[15] The ladies of the Soldiers' Relief Society of

Watkins, New York, supported Barton's work. She assured them that "every peice [*sic*] and particle [has] been given little by little to our poor suffering troops before Fredericksburg. I have more than once watched the trickling tears as they were received, and blessed you in my heart for the kindness which prompted your noble deeds. You could not have sent anything more befitting or acceptable. Your 'marmalade' as a delicacy exceeded every thing I have ever yet received—surgeons and patients sent miles for it, and the generous quantity you favored me with enabled me to gratify their wishes."[16] Welles added evangelism to his philanthropy. "We spent all of the time up to the day of the battle in visiting these regimental hospitals, supplying them with the necessaries which might otherwise have been locked up in store rooms in Washington," he recalled. "If we would bless the soldier with our bounties, let us take them to him while he is suffering on the field, give them to him in the name of Jesus, and tell him that Jesus remembers him, and would win him to the peaceful home beyond the field of strife."[17]

The days leading up to the Battle of Fredericksburg were not all work, however. The camp of the 21st Massachusetts was just a short distance from Barton's quarters, and its officers called on her frequently. Generals too dropped by to pay their respects. Inevitably, the conversation turned to the current military situation. No one seemed to agree on what Burnside's plan might be. One day the commanding general himself appeared at the house. He stood unnoticed in the doorway to Barton's room and listened while others speculated about the army's future but said nothing, a reticence that Barton found strange.[18]

CROSSING THE RAPPAHANNOCK

Burnside may have been reluctant to divulge his plans for the simple reason that he didn't have any. His entire strategy had hinged on crossing the Rappahannock River unopposed. The tardy arrival of the pontoon bridges had scuttled those plans, however, and he now found Lee's army firmly ensconced on the heights behind the town, effectively barring his way. For three weeks the Union commander pondered his options. He outnumbered Lee's army by nearly 50 percent: 115,000 to 78,000 men. Moreover, Lee had been compelled to spread his army out over a twenty-five-mile distance in order to cover the various points on the river where Burnside might attempt to cross. The Union general reasoned that if could cross the river and strike quickly, before Lee was able to concentrate his forces, he could drive the Confederates off the heights and perhaps crush a portion of their army. He chose Fredericksburg itself as his point of attack. Before dawn, December 11, Union infantry and artillery broke camp and began moving silently toward the Rappahannock where, even then, engineers were struggling to assemble the bridges without attracting the notice of Confederate pickets.

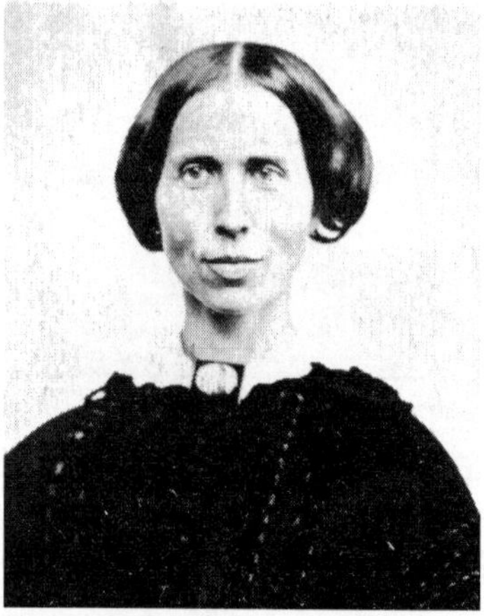

Elvira Stone, Clara Barton's cousin. (*Library of Congress*)

Meanwhile, back at the Threshley house, Clara Barton spent an uneasy night. She had heard rumors of the impending crossing and found it difficult to sleep.[19] From the solitude of her room, she penned a letter to her cousin Elvira Stone.

> My dear Cousin Vira
>
> Five minutes time with you; and God only knows what those five minutes might be worth to the-maybe-doomed thousands sleeping around me.
>
> It is the night before a battle[.] The enemy, Fredericksburg, and its mighty entrenchments lie before us, the river between,—at tomorrows dawn our troops will essay to cross, and the guns of the enemy will sweep those frail bridges at every breath.
>
> The moon is shining through the soft haze with a brightness almost prophetic. For the last half hour I have stood alone in the awful stillness of its glimmering light, gazing upon the strange sad scene around me striving to say, "Thy will Oh God be done.["]
>
> The camp fires blaze with unwonted brightness, the sentry's tread is still but quick,—the acres of little shelter tents, are dark and still, as death, no wonder for as I gazed sorrowfully upon them, I thought I could almost hear the slow flap of the grim

messenger's wings, as, one by one, he sought and selected his victims for the morning sacrifice. —Sleep weary ones. Sleep and rest for tomorrows toil. Oh! sleep and visit in dreams once more, the loved ones nestling at home. They may yet live to dream of you, cold[,] lifeless and bloody, but this dream, soldier, is thy last, paint it brightly, dream it well. Oh northern mothers[,] wives and sisters, all unconscious of the hour, would to Heaven that I could bear for you, the concentrated woe which is so soon to follow, would that Christ would teach my soul a prayer that would plead to the Father for grace sufficient for you[.] God pity and strengthen you every one.

Mine are not the only waking hours, the light yet burns brightly in our kind hearted General's tent, where he pens, what may be a last farewell to his wife and children, and thinks sadly of his fated men.

Already the roll of the moving artillery is sounding in my ears. [T]he battle draws near, and I must catch one hour's sleep for tomorrow's labor.

Good night dear cousin, and Heaven grant you strength for your more peaceful and less terrible, but not less weary days than mine[.]

Yours in love
Clara[20]

For some reason, Barton did not mail the letter for nearly three months. Its lyrical quality suggests that she may have written it with an eye toward publication.[21]

Fighting commenced shortly after daybreak when Confederate riflemen in Fredericksburg opened fire on the Union engineers attempting to span the river. Burnside responded by savagely shelling the town with 180 cannon. The sound of artillery fire awakened Barton from her troubled rest. Dressing quickly, she made her way across the fields to the Lacy House, where, from the second-story porch, she had a front-row seat of the struggle unfolding below her. "We watched (as you would watch from your own door steps a transaction in your gardens) the attempted laying down of the pontoon bridge, its abandonment under fire of the sharpshooters concealed in the cellars on the opposite bank," she wrote supporters

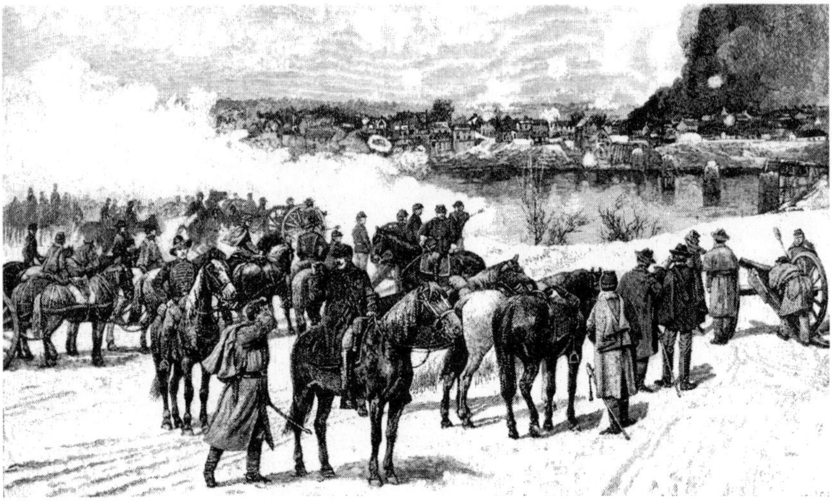

Bombardment of Fredericksburg. (*Library of Congress*)

in the North.[22] Some of the Confederate riflemen in town overshot their mark, she remembered, striking the windows and doors of the Lacy House and occasionally wounding soldiers who were standing outside.[23]

For eight hours the bombardment of Fredericksburg continued, destroying chimneys and setting buildings on fire. Still the Confederates grimly hung on. Finally, in desperation, Burnside ordered soldiers of the 7th Michigan to cross the Rappahannock in pontoon boats and wrest the town from the rebels by force. The regiment poled across the river under fire at 3 P.M., cheered on by their comrades watching from the bluffs above. Other regiments followed. At the height of the fighting, Barton pulled out her diary and scribbled herself a short note: "Capt Perkins 57th NY. Buried underneath a spice tree, on the left of the walk in front of the Lacy House. Fredericksburg is blazing in every quarter and one of the heaviest cannonades taking place which has occurred during the war. 4 oclock P.M. 11 Dec 62."[24]

Federal engineers meanwhile completed their task. Union reinforcements by the thousands pounded across the bridges and joined the fight. As darkness fell over Fredericksburg, the out-

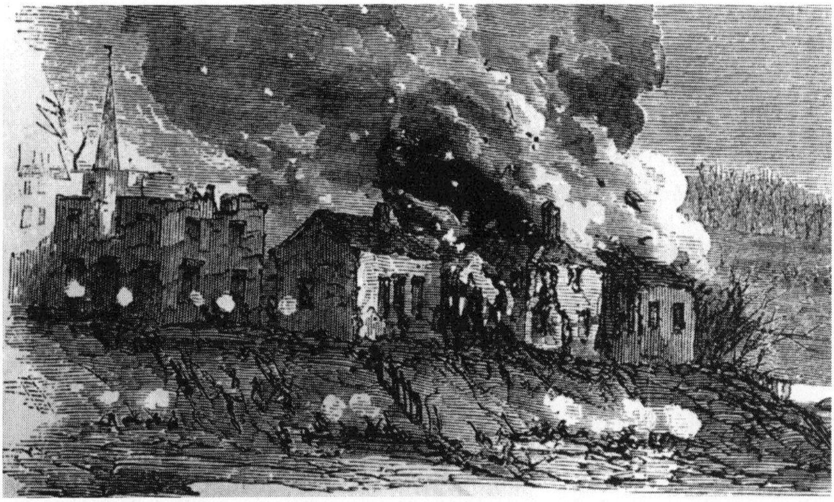

Fredericksburg under fire. (*National Park Service*)

numbered Confederates relinquished their hold on the town and fell back to their main line, three-quarters of a mile away. There, on a ridge known as Marye's Heights, they would make their stand.

THE ARMY OF THE POTOMAC'S MEDICAL DEPARTMENT

Great strides had been made in the Army of the Potomac's medical care in the months leading up to the Battle of Fredericksburg. In the summer of 1862, Dr. Jonathan Letterman became the army's medical director. Young and energetic, Letterman had overhauled the army's medical department. He created an ambulance corps operated by trained personnel and instituted a system of field hospitals organized by military divisions. Approximately twelve regiments comprised a division. Each regiment had one surgeon and one assistant surgeon. During a battle, the assistant surgeons went forward with their units, establishing aid stations a few hundred yards behind the line of battle. As wounded men came off the field, the assistant surgeons stanched their bleeding, administered anesthetics to dull their pain, and sent them to the proper division hospital in the rear.

The regimental surgeons meanwhile established division hospitals just outside the range of hostile artillery. As patients arrived from the aid stations, the surgeons made them comfortable, administered additional anesthetics, and prioritized them for treatment—much like the triage system in use today. Only the division's most capable surgeons performed operations. Each operating surgeon was supported by three assistants who restrained the patient, administered anesthesia, and otherwise assisted in the procedure. Once the operation was over, nonoperating surgeons administered additional anesthetics, set the patient aside to rest and, if he could travel, sent him to a general hospital in the North to recover. Professional pharmacists, known as hospital stewards, prescribed drugs as necessary, while musicians, convalescents, or individuals specifically detailed for the task acted as nurses.

All of these positions—surgeons, assistant surgeons, stewards, and nurses—were held by men. Women, as a rule, did not work at field hospitals, especially as early as 1862, although many, like Dorothea Dix's nurses, found employment at general hospitals well to the rear. By 1864, that would change. Women began appearing in greater numbers at the front, usually as employees of state relief agencies. In most cases, they were employed at evacuation (or depot) hospitals, where they usually prepared food for the patients, women at that time being esteemed better cooks than men. Barton differed from most other female nurses of the war in that she was not affiliated with any organization and she worked at field hospitals near the front. William E. Barton, a relative and early biographer, wrote:

> Clara Barton was more . . . than a hospital nurse. She was not simply one of a large number of women who nursed sick soldiers. She did that, hastening to assist them at the news of the very first bloodshed, and continuing until Richmond had fallen. Hers was the distinction of doing her work upon the actual field of battle; of following the cannon so as to be on the ground when the need began; of not waiting for the wounded soldier to be brought to the hospital, but of conveying the hospital to the wounded soldier. Others followed her in this good work; others accompanied her and were her faithful associates, but she was, in a very real sense, the soul and inspiration of the movement which carried comfort to wounded men while the battle was still in progress. She was not, in any narrow sense, a hospital nurse; she was, as she has justly been called, "the angel of the battlefield."[25]

THE BATTLE BEGINS IN EARNEST

Barton returned to the Threshley house on the evening of December 11, but she was back at the Lacy House early the next day establishing a kitchen and distributing supplies to the wounded.[26] It was a day of intense activity but little fighting as both sides geared up for the bloody struggle ahead. With Fredericksburg now in his possession, Burnside sent troops of Maj. Gen. Edwin V. Sumner's grand division thumping across the pontoon bridges into town while Maj. Gen. William B. Franklin's grand division crossed the Rappahannock River more than a mile downstream and deployed on the plain facing the enemy-occupied heights. In an effort to hinder the Union crossing at the pontoon bridges, Confederate batteries tossed shells, some of which landed uncomfortably close to the Lacy House. Union artillery dutifully returned the fire, Barton recalled, their blasts causing the house to quake to its very foundations.[27]

Surgeons meanwhile transformed the building into a field hospital for Brig. Gen. Oliver O. Howard's division of the Second Corps. The number of patients was still relatively small, however, and Barton had little to do. The previous day she had received a bag of apples from a little girl in the North. As the artillery thundered outside, she cut the apples into quarters and distributed them among the wounded soldiers stretched out across the house's hard wooden floors. Included in the bag was an orange. She gave it to a man who had been shot in the neck and was suffering from thirst. Holding the fruit to his mouth, she allowed the juice to trickle down his throat.[28]

The Battle of Fredericksburg reached its climax on December 13 when the Army of the Potomac launched a series of attacks against Marye's Heights, behind the town. Southern artillery and infantry repulsed the assaults with ease. Although the Confederate cannoneers directed most of their fire against the charging lines of Union infantry, they occasionally targeted Union reserves massed along the Rappahannock. "The first shots were high," recalled Barton, "crossed the river; crashed thro' our house of wounded, and fell like hail, among the reserves stationed ab[o]ut us." Harriet Eaton was with Barton at the Lacy House that day and wrote of two shells striking the building. To her diary she confided that "the noise of the musketry and cannon's roar and flash was perfectly terrific."[29] Josiah

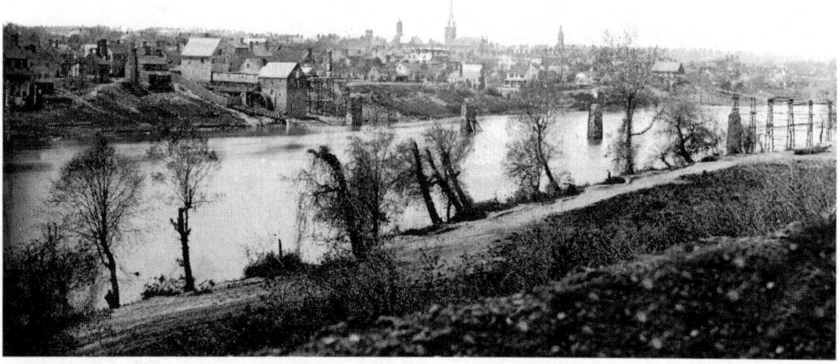

Fredericksburg. (*Library of Congress*)

F. Murphey of the 19th Massachusetts was lying wounded inside the Lacy House when a solid shot struck the building, causing it to "tremble all over. It did no damage as far as I know," he recalled, "but we held our breath expecting every minute another would come tearing through the walls and perhaps into the room where we were lying."[30] Fortunately, the day passed without any other shells striking the house, possibly because Surgeon J. Franklin Dyer had ordered a red blanket to be hung across the outside walls of the Lacy House denoting its use as a hospital. "I think they respected [it] to some extent," he wrote of the Confederates, "though a shell was thrown on Monday [December 15] into the entry next to the operating room, knocking the bricks around quite lively." Today the building exhibits no sign of damage from either bullets or shells.[31]

As the fighting across the river swelled, wounded men began arriving at the Lacy House in ever greater numbers. Among them was a man who had been struck above the ankle by a piece of shell. He was bleeding profusely. "At a glance," wrote Barton, "I discovered that an artery was severed and he was rapidly sinking. The surgeons had nearly all been ordered over into the city, and of the few who remained not one was attainable. Making a tourniquet of my handkerchief, I succeeded in arresting the flow at the first trial, gave the poor fellow some stimulant, and left him to rest and wait for better skill." Attendants placed the wounded man at the entrance to a hallway. Later, as Barton passed back and forth between rooms, the man snatched at the hem of her dress. "He could not speak aloud,'" she wrote, "but the tears were sliding quietly down his brown, dust-covered cheeks. As I knelt to learn his wishes, he whispered faintly, 'You saved my life.'" According to Barton, this happened several times over the course of the next few days. Each time the man whispered the same four words, "You saved my life." Months later, as she was sifting through some papers at her Washington, D.C., residence, there was a knock at her door. "I hastened to open it," she wrote, "and there, leaning upon his crutch, stood my hero of the *four words,* and before I could recover from my surprise sufficiently to speak, he broke silence with, '*You saved my life.*'" Curiously, Barton did not record the soldier's name.[32]

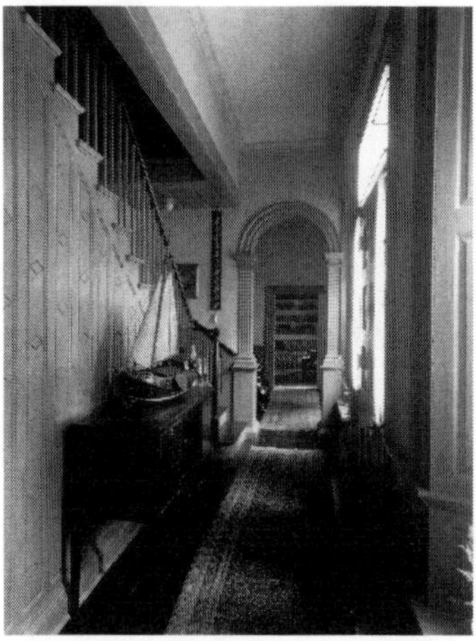

One of the Lacy House hallways as it appeared in the 1920s. (*Library of Congress*)

IN THE TOWN

At a point early in the battle, a courier dashed up the steps of the Lacy House and delivered into Barton's hands a scribbled note that read, "We want more liquors & something to Eat. Your place is here. Hundreds of wounded men & but few to work. Come." Barton later remembered the note as having been written by a surgeon in the town, but it was actually penned by her assistant, Cornie Welles, who had crossed the river ahead of her. Today the note, containing Welles's signature, is among the Clara Barton Papers at the Library of Congress.[33] When Barton's teamsters learned the nature of her summons, she wrote that their faces "grew ashy white . . . and the lips which had cursed and scowled in disgust trembled as they begged me to send *them* but *save myself*. I could only permit them to go *with* me if they chose," Barton wrote, "and in 20 minutes we were rocking across the swaying bridge, the water hissing with shot on either side."[34]

According to one of Barton's early biographers, a wounded Confederate officer overheard the conversation. Summoning Barton to his side, he confided to her that Fredericksburg was a death trap and urged her not to enter the town. "Every street and lane of the city is covered by our cannon," he explained. "They are now concealed, and do not reply to the bombardment of your army, because they wish to entice you across. When your entire army has reached the other side of the Rappahannock and attempts to move along the streets, they will find Fredericksburg only a slaughter pen, and not a regiment of them will be allowed to escape. Do not go over, for you will go to certain death!" Barton appreciated the soldier's kindness but she disregarded his warning. She was determined to go where needed.[35]

Barton herself never mentioned this unlikely incident, and it probably never took place. If it did, it may have been Capt. Thomas W. Thurman of the 13th Mississippi who gave her the warning. Thurman had been wounded in Fredericksburg on December 11 and was taken back to the Lacy House, where he remained for several days, chatting freely with Northern soldiers and civilians alike. That Clara Barton spoke with Thurman at some point is certain, for she jotted his name down in her diary.[36]

Barton hurried down the slope leading to the river and crossed on one of the swaying bridges. At the western end, an officer stepped forward to help her onto the shore. She later told crowds that "While our hands were raised in the act of stepping down a piece of an exploding shell hissed thro' between us, just below our arms, carrying away a portion of both the skirts of his coat and my dress, ricocheting along the ground a few rods from us like a harmless pebble upon the water. The next instant a solid shot thundered over our heads, a noble steed bounded in air and with his gallant rider rolled in the dirt not 30 feet in the rear. Leaving the kind-hearted officer, I passed on alone to the hospital. In less than a half hour he was bro[ugh]t to me dead." Lest her audience interpret her story as boasting, she hastily added: "I mention these circumstances *not* as

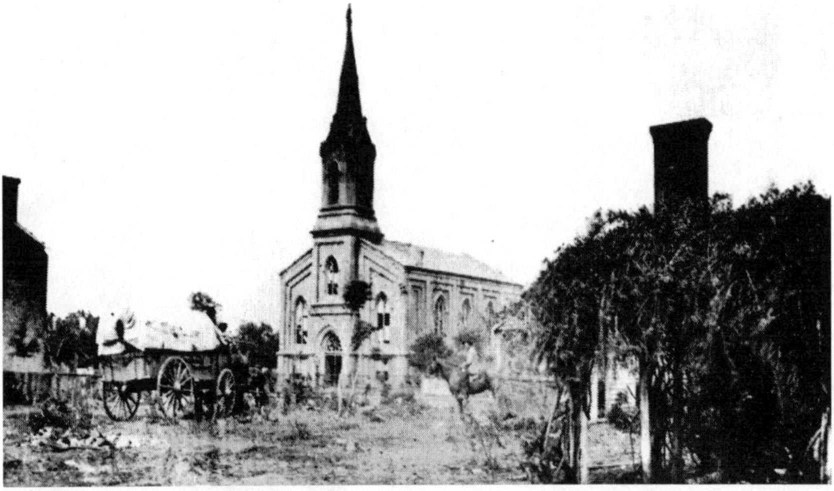

Fredericksburg Baptist Church. (*Library of Congress*)

specimens of my own bravery. *Oh! no,* I beg you will not place *that* construction upon it, for I never professed anything beyond ordinary courage and a thousand times prefer safety to danger."[37]

Once in town, Barton joined Welles at a field hospital supervised by her friend Surgeon Calvin Cutter of the 21st Massachusetts, who was then serving as medical director of Sturgis's division.[38] Cutter had established hospitals in six of the town structures: the Baptist church, the orphans' asylum, and four private dwellings.[39] Barton appears to have worked at a house near the church, where, according to an early biographer, she "at once organized hospital kitchens, provided supplies for the wounded, and when the wounded men were brought in, sought to alleviate their sufferings."[40] "We received the first who were brought off the field, and assisted in dressing their ghastly wounds," wrote Welles. "All through that afternoon and night the wounded were being brought into the city, and as well cared for as was possible under the circumstances."[41]

During the day Barton moved among the different buildings, dodging in and out among the regiments headed for Marye's Heights. Being alone and one of the few women present that day, she attracted the notice of Brig. Gen. Marsena R. Patrick, the army's provost marshal. Believing Barton to be a resident of the town, Patrick

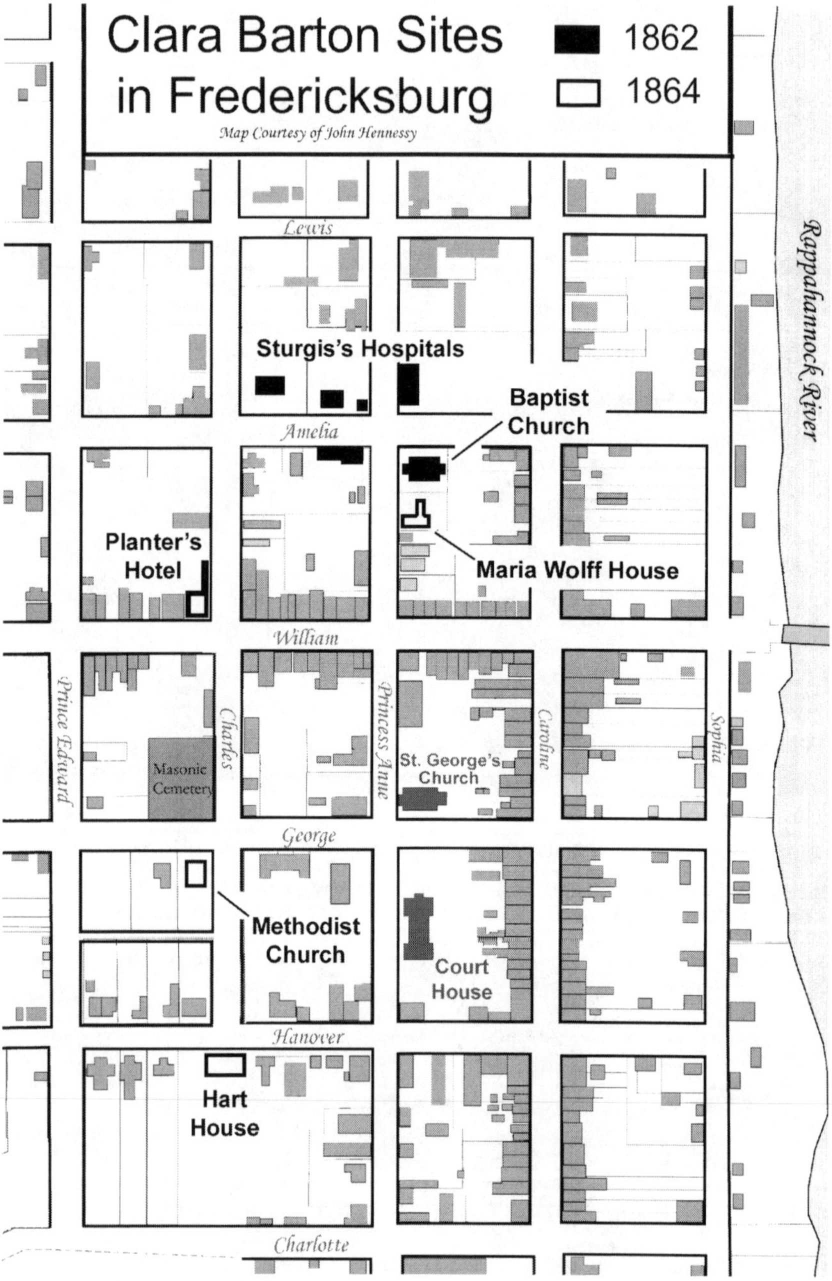

Clara Barton sites in Fredericksburg, 1862 and 1864. (John Hennessy)

galloped over to her and said kindly, "You are alone and in great danger, madam. Do you want protection?" "Amused at his gallant mistake," wrote Barton, "I humored it by thanking him as I turned to the ranks and adding that I believed myself to be the best protected women in the United States. The soldiers nearest me caught my words and responding with 'that's so, that's so,' set up a cheer. This, in turn, was caught by the next line and so on, line after line, till the whole army joined in the shout, no one knowing what he was cheering at but never doubting there was victory somewhere. The gallant old general, taking in the situation, bowed low his bared head, saying, as he galloped away, 'I believe you are right, madam.'"[42]

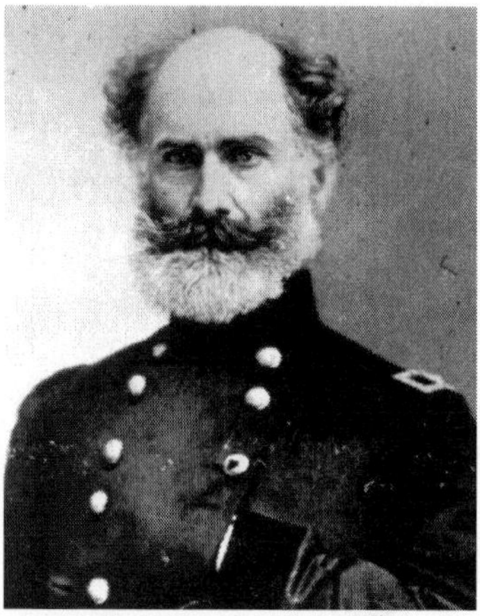

General Marsena Patrick. (*National Archives*)

General Patrick kept a detailed diary of his Civil War experiences, but he wrote nothing of this singular incident, suggesting that it made little impression upon him. In all likelihood, Barton took what was a routine encounter and inflated it into an episode of heroic proportions. That passing soldiers would be able to hear her comments over the din of battle is unlikely. That they would pause in the midst of their advance to cheer her is preposterous.[43] Correspondent Charles Page of the *New York Tribune* saw Barton moving through the crowded streets and expected every moment to see her shot. He witnessed the encounter between Barton and Patrick and recalled that the general remonstrated with her about remaining in the town. In his conversation with Barton, Page said nothing about the troops cheering her, or if he did, Barton did not record it.[44]

Meanwhile, the 21st Massachusetts was suffering one of its worst days of the war. The regiment had crossed the Rappahannock with 284 men. On December 13, it went forward to support the picket line of another division and by the end of the day had lost eight men killed, fifty-six wounded, and five missing—nearly one-quarter of its force.[45] Barton was nearly a mile away from the regiment and in a different part of town when it attacked. Claims that she watched anxiously as it waded into battle have no basis in fact.[46]

Barton and Welles passed among the wounded men, giving them food and offering whatever assistance they could. "Many instances of bravery came under our notice," wrote Welles. "One of the wounded exclaimed, as news came that we were driving the rebels, 'Glory! I am willing to die now,' and immediately expired. One noble young officer, suffering much from his wound, said, as I passed a piece of bread and butter to him, 'Perhaps some of the boys need it more than I.' 'I have plenty for all,' said I. 'Then I will eat it,'" he replied. Welles remembered that his female companion too showed uncommon courage that day. "One shell shattered the door of the room in which Miss Barton was attending to wounded men," he wrote. "True to her mission, she did not flinch, but continued her duties as usual." This would not have surprised Lt. Col. John Elwell, who characterized Barton as being "insensible to fear."[47]

Barton remained in Fredericksburg on December 14. At one point in the day, an officer rushed up to her and excitedly explained that one of his soldiers had been shot in the face. Blood from the wound had dried in his mouth and nose and was cutting off his supply of air. Would Barton come help him? Seizing a basin of water and a sponge, she hurried across the street. Inside the crowded sanctuary she found the man, his face encased in blood. "For any human appearance above the shoulders it might as well have been any thing else as a man," she later recalled. "neither *sight*, nor *speech*, no *flesh* visible." Barton knelt by the man's side and gingerly began removing the dried blood. For a half hour she labored, all the while fearing that the hemorrhaging might resume and cause the man to suffocate. Little by little, a face began to emerge. To Barton's surprise, the features seemed familiar. "Finally my hand wiped away the last obstruction. An eye opened, and there to my gaze was the sexton of my own old home church."[48] Barton continued to wipe away the blood, and the man—Pvt. Nathan P. Rice of the 21st Massachusetts—survived.[49] Military records confirm that Rice was shot in the face at Fredericksburg and was discharged as a result of his wound on February 28, 1863.[50]

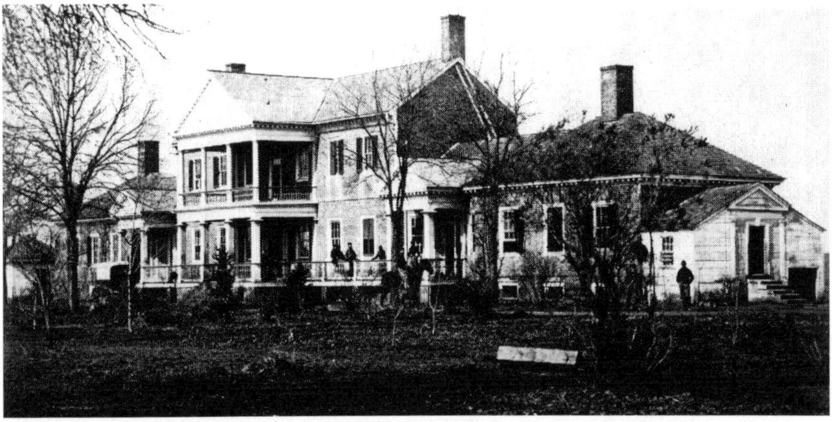

The Lacy House. (*Library of Congress*)

RETURN TO THE LACY HOUSE

The defeat at Fredericksburg prompted Burnside to retreat, and on the night of December 15–16 the Army of the Potomac quietly fell back across the Rappahannock River to its former camps in Stafford County. Darkness and rain concealed the retreat from the enemy, and the movement was attended without significant loss. Rather than remain with the wounded men of Sturgis's division, Barton returned to the Lacy House and its "fearful scenes." It was a strange decision, given her close association with Sturgis and his division.[51]

By then the Lacy House had become a scene of terrible suffering and death. Barton found the building packed upstairs and down with soldiers exhibiting grievous wounds of every description. "They covered every foot of the floors and porticos," she later told her audiences, and "lay on the stair landings. A man who could find opportunity to lie between the legs of a table thought himself rich; *he* was not likely to be stepped on. In a common cupboard with four shelves 5 men lay and were fed and attended. 3 lived to be removed and 2 died of their wounds. Think of trying to lie still and die quietly lest you fall out of a bed six feet high."[52]

Barton's description of patients being stacked like china on the cupboard shelves of the Lacy House defies credibility, as does her estimate that 1,200 wounded men simultaneously occupied the building, a figure roughly equal to 120 patients per room.[53] Surgeon

J. Franklin Dyer, who was in charge of the hospital, set a more reasonable figure. On December 18, he informed his wife: "We have about two hundred here now and have had all the time, some coming over the bridges, and some going all the time." Even at just 200 patients, the building was packed. "I have the house full," he wrote, "men lie on the floors as close as they can be stowed, a little straw here and there; the best we can do for them."[54]

When the house became full, Dyer erected six large tents on the lawn, each capable of holding ten men. The canvas shelters had no source of heat and at nights became frigid. Stoves arrived on December 20, a week after the battle. In the meantime, Barton alleviated the patients' suffering by building large fires, wrapping the men in blankets, and having her assistants heat bricks from a collapsed chimney and place them around the shivering men. Hot drinks and pallets made of pine boughs and quilts added to the freezing soldiers' relief.[55]

On or before December 18, Surgeon General Albert Hammond journeyed to the Lacy House to see for himself the care being afforded to the wounded soldiers. A number of medical inspectors and Congressmen accompanied him, among them Barton's patron and friend Senator Henry Wilson. Earlier in the year, Hammond had given Barton 130 gallons of confiscated liquor for distribution among the troops. She distributed some of it to thirty-three badly wounded soldiers who had just come into Union lines under a flag of truce and to others struggling with pain—enough, thought Linus Brockett, to make them all "measurably drunk."[56]

Barton labored at the Lacy House for the next two weeks. During the day she prepared food for the soldiers in the plantation's detached kitchen, and at night she slept in a tent encircled by her small train of wagons.[57] Headstrong and inflated by a sense of her own importance, Barton inevitably clashed with the hospital staff. She plagued Surgeon J. Franklin Dyer to such a degree that he finally ordered her out of the kitchen and put one of his own men in charge of it. The following year, when he learned that Barton had gone to South Carolina, he expressed a fervent desire that she would stay there—or at least not return to the Army of the Potomac. Other surgeons in the army may have echoed the sentiment.[58]

Unaware, perhaps, of his companion's conflicts with the authorities, Welles went about the business of providing physical comfort to the living and spiritual comfort to the dying. He viewed himself as a representative of Christ. "Many were brought to our hospital naked, and we clothed them"; wrote Welles,

> the greater portion were very hungry; and some nearly famished—we fed them. Many were exhausted with bleeding wounds—we staunched and bound up their wounds, and revived them with cordials. We provided pillows for hundreds of broken and amputated limbs. We fed several hundreds of wounded men for a number of days from our kitchen, manned by seven men. Our kitchen was furnished and bountifully supplied by kind friends at the North. In many instances, in place of loved ones at home, have we wiped the cold damps of death from the brow, while we could breathe a word of prayer that they might have the consolations of him whose presence in such dying hours is life, health and peace.[59]

During the two weeks that she was at the Lacy House, Barton had an opportunity to talk with many of the wounded soldiers. She jotted down the names of twenty-six men that she met there, including at least three Confederates.[60] First Lieutenant Edgar M. Newcomb was a particularly sad case. The twenty-two-year-old Harvard graduate had enlisted in the 19th Massachusetts as a corporal and had been twice promoted for gallantry. In the attacks on Marye's Heights, he had picked up the flag of a fallen color-bearer only to have a bullet, or perhaps a shell fragment, slice through the calves of both his legs. As he crumpled to earth, he handed the cherished banner to a fellow officer, admonishing him not to let the flag touch the ground. Two friends later rescued Newcomb from the field and sent him to the rear, but it was clear that his days were numbered.[61]

Barton found the young man hemorrhaging in a bedroom on the upper floor of the Lacy House. His brother, Charlie, was at his side. Barton occasionally sat with Charlie and joined him in quietly singing hymns and quoting scripture to his dying brother. When in his delirium Edgar imagined Barton to be his mother, she "kindly favored the illusion by shading the light," a fellow officer recalled, just as she had done with Hugh Johnson at Fairfax Station. The young lieutenant succumbed to his injuries before dawn on December 20 with Barton, his brother, and a soldier of his regiment at his side. Barton later wrote an acquaintance: "When I rose from the side of the couch where I had knelt for hours, until the last breath had faded, I wrung the blood from the bottom of my clothing before I could step, for the weight about my feet. Dreadful days, dear Sister . . . one's heart grows sick to think of it."[62]

Another memorable patient was young Wriley Faulkner of the 7th Michigan, who had been shot through the lungs on December 11 during the initial assault on the town. Male nurses found a spot for him in the corner of a room. Certain that he would die, Barton wrote down the young man's name and address, perhaps with the intention of contacting his parents later on, but Faulkner surprised everyone by stubbornly clinging to life. After several days at the Lacy House, he was wrapped in a blanket and sent off to Lincoln General Hospital in Washington. As he departed, Barton handed him a bottle of milk punch for nourishment.[63]

Barton was particularly drawn to Sgt. Thomas Plunkett. When the 21st Massachusetts's flag fell to the ground in the assault against Marye's Heights, Plunkett seized the fallen banner and carried it forward until an exploding shell tore away both of his forearms. Miraculously, he survived the ordeal and made it back to the Lacy House. When she heard of the sergeant's heroic conduct, Barton took a special interest in his welfare. She later used her influence with Senator Wilson to get Plunkett a furlough and secure for him a substantial pension. He later received the Medal of Honor for his actions.[64]

By the final week of December most of the wounded soldiers at the Lacy House had been taken to Falmouth Station and placed aboard trains for Aquia Landing. From there, steamboats transported them to general hospitals in the North. Using what was left of Hammond's liquor, Barton made hot toddies for the soldiers to take with them on their journey.[65] Plunkett was among the last to leave. On Christmas Day, strong arms hoisted his stretcher onto a train at Falmouth Station. Barton and some of Plunkett's comrades in the 21st Massachusetts saw him off.[66] Barton herself returned to Washington later that week. She had been away from home for more than a month, and when she entered her apartment on New Year's Eve she was both physically and emotionally spent.[67] She later recalled her feelings at the time: "The fires of *Fredericksburg* still blazed before my eyes, and her cannon still thundered at my ear, while away down in the depths of my heart I was smothering the groans and treasuring the prayers of her dead and dying heroes,—worn, weak, and heart sick, I was *home from Fredericksburg*; and when, there, for the first time I looked at myself, shoeless, gloveless, ragged and bloodstained, a new sense of desolation and pity, and sympathy and weariness all blended swept over me with irresistible force, and, perfectly overpowered, I sank down . . . and wept as I had never done since."[68]

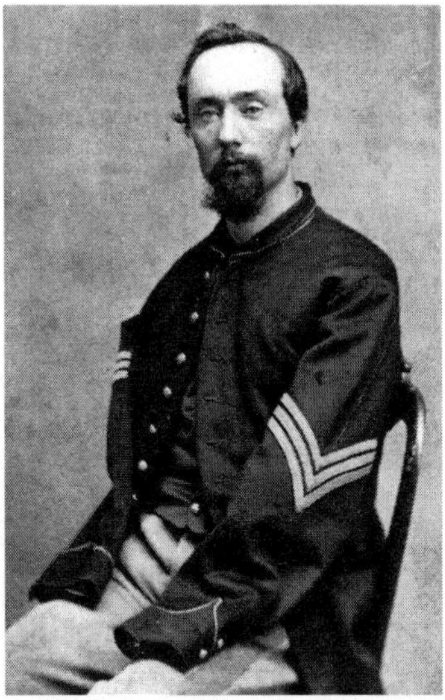

Sergeant Thomas Plunkett. (*Massachusetts MOLLUS Collection*)

She had been at home for three months when a messenger from Lincoln Hospital appeared at her door with a note that the men in Ward 17 wished to see her. "I returned with him," Barton later told audiences, "and as I entered the ward 70 men saluted me, standing, such as could, others rising feebly in their beds and falling back, exhausted with the effort. Every man had left his blood in Fredericksburg. Every one was from the Lacy House. My hand had dressed every wound, many of them in the first terrible moments of agony. I had prepared their food in the snow and winds of December and fed them like children. How *dear* they had grown to me in their sufferings, and the 3 great cheers that greeted my entrance into that hospital ward were dearer than the applause that sounded sweeter than the voice of Josephine." When the ovation subsided, a young man stepped forward and, extending his hand, announced: "I am Wriley Faulkner of the 7th Michigan. I didn't die and the milk punch lasted all the way to Washington!"[69]

4

Months of Frustration

"THE WORLD APPEARED SELFISH AND TREACHEROUS"

Upon her return from Falmouth, Barton caught up on lapsed correspondence and amassed supplies for her next campaign. She still had much to do, however, when her friend, Col. Rucker, sent her word that the Army of the Potomac was preparing to launch a mid-winter campaign across the Rappahannock. Within twelve hours she was on a ship heading back to Aquia Landing, accompanied by Cornie Welles and a Mr. J. W. Doe of Massachusetts. Barton's nephew, Sam, noted that before she left Washington, Rucker "gave her two new tents, and bread, flour, meal, and a new stove." He insisted that she "telegraph to him for anything she wanted and he would send it to her."[1]

Barton and her associates reached Falmouth on the night of January 18, 1863, to find the army under marching orders. Two days later, William B. Franklin's and Joseph Hooker's grand divisions broke camp and started for Banks's Ford, a shallow point on the Rappahannock just a few miles above Fredericksburg. Burnside's luck was no better in January than it had been in December, however, and before his troops could cross the river the weather, which to that

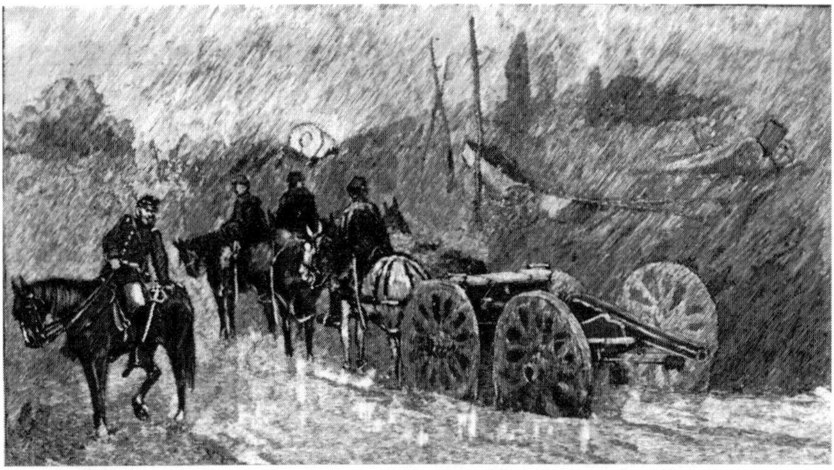

The Mud March. (*Warren Goss*, Recollections of a Private)

point had been unseasonably pleasant, turned ugly. Wind and rain lashed the countryside, transforming the unpaved clay roads into ribbons of thick, clinging mud. To Barton, who remained hunkered down at Falmouth with Sumner's troops, it seemed like "the stormiest night I ever knew."[2] The rain continued to beat down upon the countryside without remission the next day. On January 22, with the river overflowing its banks and his troops hopelessly mired in the slough, Burnside ordered the army back to its winter camps. The Mud March, as it came to be known, was over.[3]

Barton returned to Washington as soon as the campaign ended. Before departing, she distributed 120 pairs of mittens made by the ladies of Worcester for the men of the 21st Massachusetts, who were then on picket duty at the Lacy House. She returned to Falmouth briefly on February 3 to retrieve some supplies; otherwise, she spent the winter months in the nation's capital.[4] In later years, however, she asserted that she spent the entire winter with the army. In a speech delivered in January 1888, Barton declared that she "remained till nearly spring with the sick and wounded in the field—about 7 months." Moreover, she insisted that she was "never under a roof at night that winter & the snow sometimes 2 ft. deep."[5] This is patently false. Letters written by her in the early months of 1863 clearly indicate that she wintered in Washington.[6]

Many of the letters she wrote that winter were addressed to individuals or organizations that supported her work. It was a tedious but necessary part of the job, and Barton was good at it. She made her benefactors feel that they were more than simply coworkers with her in a glorious enterprise; they were her personal friends. Her letters stressed how important their gifts were and how much both she and the soldiers appreciated them.[7] Such missives became more critical as the war progressed and Barton found herself competing for donations with nationwide organizations such as the United States Christian and Sanitary Commissions.

THE DEPARTMENT OF THE SOUTH

With the arrival of spring Barton returned to the field, but she went to South Carolina rather than Virginia. In February 1863 the Ninth Corps left the Army of the Potomac and headed west, taking with it the 21st Massachusetts. With her hometown regiment no longer in Virginia, she elected to accompany her brother David to Hilton Head, South Carolina, where Union troops were preparing for a campaign against Charleston. Barton had used her influence with Wilson to have David appointed a captain in the Quartermaster Corps, a position advantageous to Clara in that it would give her ready access to the army larder and possibly provide her a protector when she was in the field. She apparently did this without David's knowledge or consent. She hoped that the army would assign him to the Army of the Potomac, but instead he received orders to report to Hilton Head. The assignment pleased neither David nor his family. According to Clara, her brother held her "responsible for placing him in a position entirely new to him, and his family held me responsible for his personal safety in a deadly climate and insisted upon my accompanying him." Clara reluctantly agreed to go. "I left all and went with him," she wrote a year later in self-pity, "smoothed every rough path for him.—he walked on the roses, and I trampled the thorns the whole year." Ironically, except for a few weeks that she spent on Morris Island, the experience in South Carolina more closely resembled a vacation than work.[8]

Clara and David arrived in Hilton Head aboard the U.S.S. *Arago* on April 7, the very day Union ironclads attacked Fort Sumter in

Charleston harbor.[9] The attack failed miserably and the ships returned to Port Royal, twelve miles from Hilton Head. While Union commanders devised a new strategy for capturing Charleston, Clara and her brother settled into a house on the island. Like most of the buildings constructed by the army there, the house was long and low with pine floors. She and David occupied adjoining rooms in the house, each fourteen feet square in size, with three closets, two fireplaces, and two windows, the latter dressed with mosquito netting. Pieces confiscated from local houses comprised the furnishings. Clara's room, which also served as a parlor, contained a bed, a rocking chair upholstered with crimson damask, a cane chair, and a stuffed black chair. In addition, she had her trunk, which doubled as a safe, a large solid mahogany table trimmed in brass that stood underneath one of the windows, and a large center table made of black Egyptian marble. "Now picture to yourself the grotesque appearance of such a suite of rooms, and then think of entertaining therein Company of the highest order of intellect and accustomed to all the luxuries of social life, from private soldiers to Major Generals," she laughingly suggested to her cousin Elvira Stone.[10]

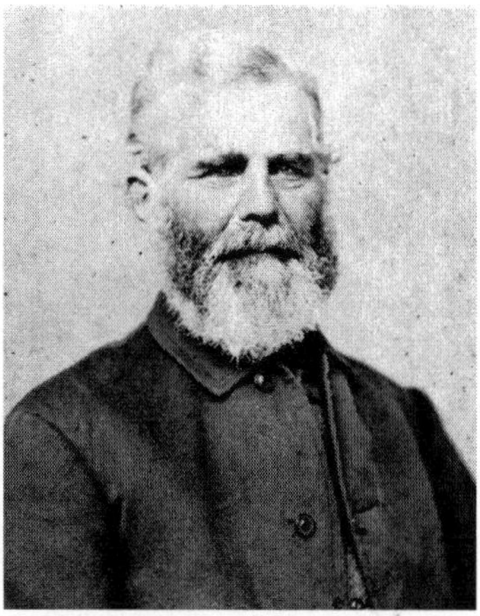
David Barton. (*Library of Congress*)

For three months Barton had little to do but enjoy the coastal scenery and socialize with the Department of the South's officers, most notably Lt. Col. John Elwell, the department's chief quartermaster, and Capt. Samuel T. Lamb, the depot quartermaster. She entertained guests at her house each day, took frequent rides with Elwell, Lamb, and others along the beach, and made occasional trips to nearby islands. It was an idyllic life, especially in wartime, but it lacked excitement and purpose. After a few weeks Barton grew tired of it all and found herself longing to return to action.[11]

She would soon get her chance. Having failed to reduce Fort Sumter with naval power, the department commander, Maj. Gen. Quincy A. Gillmore, decided to erect batteries on Morris Island, at the mouth of Charleston harbor, and pound the fort into submission. In the way stood a small Confederate fort called Battery Wagner. On July 10, Union troops unsuccessfully attacked the fort and suffered heavy casualties. Barton witnessed the assault from the deck of a ship anchored offshore. The single discharge of a Union cannon just after dawn signaled the start of the attack. Soon dozens of guns were in play, their bursting shells striking the parapet of the Confederate fort and throwing sand 50 feet into the air. Barton watched, transfixed, as Union infantry waded ashore. "lo! our troop[s] were leaping from the boats like wildcats, and scarce waiting to form, on they went, in one wild Charge, across the marsh and up the banks, and onto the entrenchments," she wrote to Elvira later in the day, "and almost in a breath, up rose the *Old Flag*, and the ground was ours, with from fifty to a hundred prisoners from almost under the *guns of Sumpter*." Within moments, however, the fort's guns responded, unleashing a torrent of shot and shell on the sand battery. "Red spouts of fire, hissing balls, and columns of smoke towering to the skies poured forth inces[s]ently," she recalled. The federal soldiers fell back a few hundred yards and began throwing up breastworks across the beach.[12]

The next morning, the federals renewed their assault. The 7th Connecticut led the charge followed by the 9th Maine and 76th Pennsylvania. The men from the Nutmeg State gallantly clawed their way up the outside face of the fort's sandy wall but had to relinquish their gains when the trailing regiments failed to come promptly to their support. Again, the Union army had to fall back. Recriminations followed. "Of course, as our forces did not succeed upon the *first trial in going entirely through the enemies works some one* must be very much to blame," commented Barton, "or Madame Rumor would be untrue to her vocation. The blame is thrown first upon one, and then the other, of the two supporting regiments, but *I* am more inclined to the belief that the difficulty consisted in the vulnerable and perishable nature of flesh and blood, as compared with lead and iron."[13]

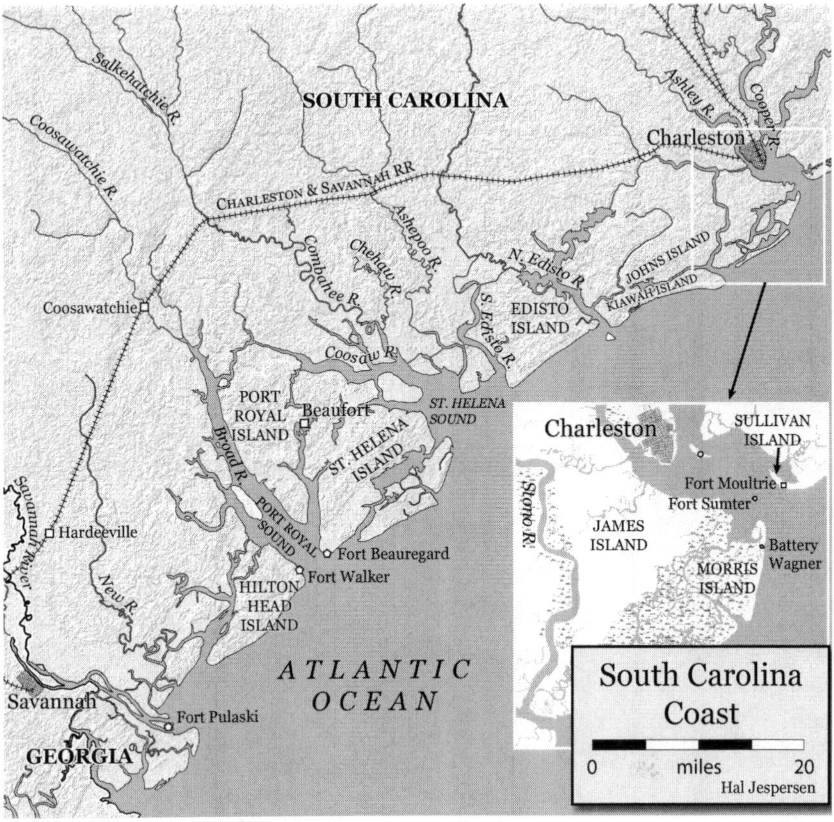

Clara Barton sites in South Carolina.

Gillmore refused to admit defeat. Still convinced he could capture the fort by direct assault, he ferried additional men and guns over to the island and renewed the attack on July 18. By then, Barton had joined the troops massing on the island, bringing with her an ambulance, horses, driver, and saddle horse, but few supplies.[14] "My tent stands with the front hospital, a mile and a half below Fort Wagner, just on the beach," she informed a cousin, "a slight bluff, on the top of which we are, holds back the breakers which roll and dash at us incessantly,—directly up the beach to our left, as we face the sea, is Fort Wagner, before which our troops are fortifying and entrenching with incredible speed." Just out to sea, on her right,

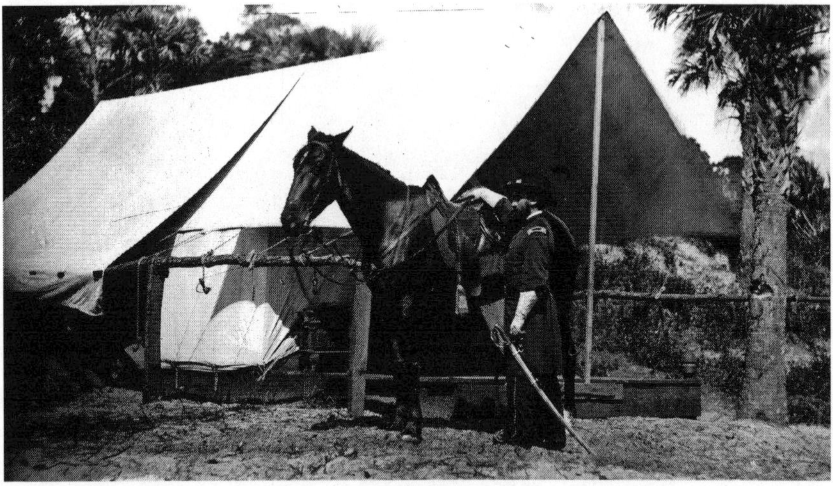
General Quincy Gillmore on Morris Island. (*Library of Congress*)

stood the fleet of the Southern Atlantic Blockading Squadron, headed by the armor-plated U.S.S. *New Ironsides*; General Gillmore's flagship, the *Mary Benton*; and the turreted monitor *Canonicus*. Also part of the squadron was the U.S.S. *Philadelphia*, the ship on which Barton resided when she was not ashore.[15]

Barton watched Gillmore's July 18 attack on Battery Wagner from a high point on Morris Island called Lookout Hill. Like the earlier attacks, she found the sight "grand beyond description." To Annie Childs she wrote: "The flash of a hundred guns and ten thousand muskets lit up the darkness of our desert island, and the thunders of Wagner and 'Sumpter' shook it to its center; and on those bloody 'parapets' freedom and slavery met and wrestled hand to hand, and the [rebel] flag and the true swelling in the same breeze stood face to face while warriors met and fought, and martyrs died; through the long, dark terrible hours, we gazed and hoped and prayed, and at length—must I write it?—turned back in despair to comfort our wounded and bury our dead. Repulsed!!" Although later sources insist that she risked her life succoring wounded soldiers who lay within two hundred yards of the fort, Barton says nothing of such heroics either in her diary or in her letter to Childs. Had she done so, she certainly would have mentioned it. She did pitch in after the fact, however, preparing food for the wounded, covering them with blankets, and helping them to board hospital ships.[16]

Having failed to take Battery Wagner by direct assault, Gillmore decided to dig approaches to the fort and level it with artillery. Over the next ten weeks, his trenches and guns crept ever closer to the parapet. Recognizing the hopelessness of their situation, the Confederates abandoned the sand battery on September 7, slipping away under cover of darkness. Gillmore was now free to train his artillery on Fort Sumter itself. For weeks his big guns pounded the fort, located in the center of the channel, but ironically the more they reduced its brick walls to rubble the stronger it became. The federals would not capture Sumter, nor Charleston, for another year and a half, and only then because the enemy abandoned it.

Meanwhile, troops on both sides had to endure constant, if desultory, shelling. "Not an inch of that Island in my opinion but lies under fire of the enemies batteries," Barton explained to Stone. "Frequently shells burst at night within 1/4 of a mile of my tent, and no hour of the night that the cannon did not thunder in our ears. although one may care very little for these things and they become like an every day tale still they wear a little upon the rest even of our hardiest soldiers because you cannot forget the fact that possibly each shot as it falls upon your ears has sent some poor fellow to the earth w[r]ithing in agony."[17] Barton saw them all: a German immigrant who had lost his leg, another soldier missing a left hand, a third with a crushed left leg and a broken right leg. When it came to cannonballs, there were few minor injuries.[18]

One of Barton's most illustrious patients was Lt. Col. Robert Leggett of the 10th Connecticut, who, she reported, "was commanding his men in the trenches, when a shot came hitting his sword, cutting his leg *completely* off—just below the knee."[19] According to John Elwell, Barton immediately went to Leggett's relief, "dropped by his side, hurri[e]dly tore off some of her apparel, bound the torn limb, improvised a tourniquet, holding tight the bleeding fragments until a surgeon could amputate the limb."[20] Despite the operation, few believed Leggett would survive. Surgeons tried to get him to take some stimulants, but he refused to do so until Barton gently persuaded him to submit. After that, the doctors were

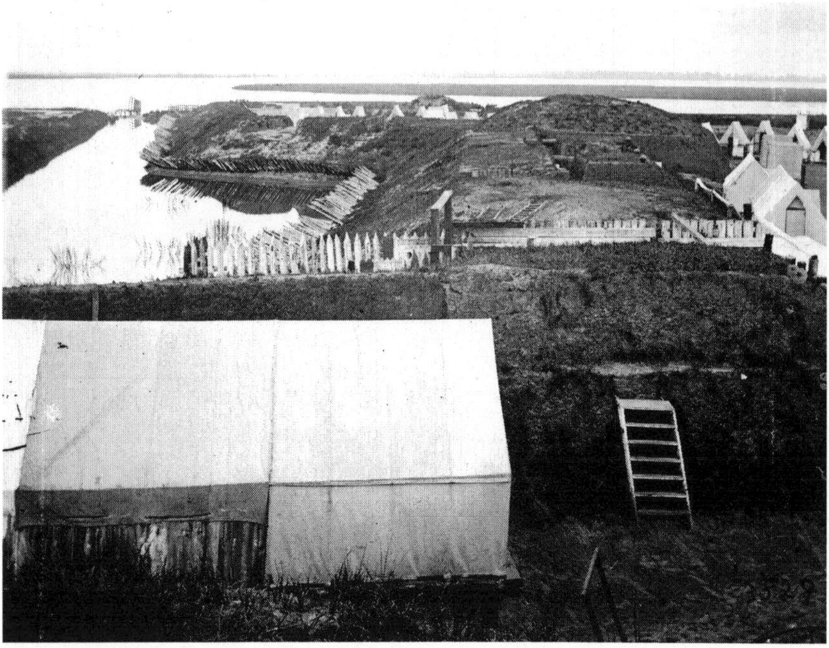

Battery Wagner as it appeared in 1865. (*Library of Congress*)

content to let her manage him. "I talked cheerfully with him told him it was a small loss to lose a leg," she recalled. "He could go into the field again in a few months." With Barton's encouragement Leggett revived, enabling surgeons to operate on his leg. Afterward, they moved him to a spot near Barton's tent, where she could personally keep an eye on him. Under her care, he became "one of the most contented happy fellows I ever saw—playful as a child," wrote his nurse, even though infection had set in, giving him chills and fever. Leggett's patience amid suffering reminded Barton very much of her brother David, whom she had nursed to health as a child. "I have thought of you so many times when I have stood over him shaking," she told her brother, "and then the poor and drenching sweat all night after and still he makes no complaint. . . . I think our soldiers are brave and patient men,—worth taking care of—and worth feeding."[21] Leggett survived his wound and in gratitude for Barton's care would later name a daughter after her.[22]

Another prominent officer wounded on Morris Island was Col. Alvin C. Voris of the 67th Ohio, who was shot in the lower abdomen on July 18 while leading his regiment in an attack on Battery Wagner. John Elwell later claimed that he saw Barton rescue Voris, but neither patient nor nurse ever made such a claim. On the contrary, Barton later told Voris that she saw him on the night of his wounding, but he was asleep and she thought it best to let him rest." Voris recovered from his injury and would encounter Barton again in Virginia, where the two became fast friends.[23]

Barton remained on Morris Island for several weeks following the assault on Battery Wagner. She made her quarters near Lighthouse Inlet among the tents of Surgeon John J. Craven's "advance hospital." Although located at the extreme southern end of the island, farthest from Sumter, the hospital was nonetheless subject to frequent shelling, so much so that Barton felt it prudent to keep her personal trunks aboard the U.S.S. *Philadelphia*. In addition to her tent, the army issued Barton an ambulance, horses, and driver to use while on the island, plus a saddle horse for her own personal needs.[24] She provided pillows and blankets for the soldiers from her private stores as well as special dietary items such as fruit, porridge, dried milk, and eggs. Although she probably ate the same food as her patients, when she described the hardships she had suffered on Morris Island to her friend Senator Wilson less than a year later, she wrote of eating moldy hardtack and drinking brackish water.[25]

Food and drink aside, it was not an easy life. With only moderate exaggeration, she later recalled being "scorched by the sun, chilled by the waves, rocked by the tempest, buried in the shifting sand, toiling day after day in the trenches." Barton's cousin Leander Poor saw the hardship firsthand. "To *think* of establishing one's self in range of hostile guns, and administering comfort to the wounded and solace to the dying may be romantic," he wrote his aunt Elvira Stone, "but requires the heart and nerve that Clara alone of a thousand possess to calmly meet the stern realities that heap themselves, like thorns in the pathway of the angel of the battlefield. One can form nothing like a correct idea of the horrors of the field hospital in the day of battle, unless he has been a present witness."[26]

Barton's health eventually gave way under the brutal conditions. After about four weeks on the island, she contracted what she described as a "slight disease" and returned to Hilton Head. Although she made light of her condition, Poor considered it "very severe" and believed she would not recover. Barton herself admitted that she barely escaped with her life. "I[,] no longer able to see, was lying weak and helpless as a child, little knowing and less minding towards what goal my way was wending," she later confessed. After several weeks of rest, however, she pulled through, and by the end of August she was again clamoring to return to Morris Island. "I have learned to labor, and chafe at *rest*, while our men suffer and die," she informed Stone, "but I must wait and watch and hope, and bide my time."[27] She finally got her wish on September 7, the very day Battery Wagner fell to Union arms. In contrast to July, when she "had but few supplies and few conveniences for preparing them for issue," she now came laden with foodstuffs and stores of every description. "She has spacious tents awaiting her," wrote Poor, "and is to be attended by an intelligent colored woman whom we call *Aunt Betty*, or *Aunty*."[28]

Barton's friends in the department arranged to have her tent placed in rear of the hospital and detailed a fatigue party to level the ground. But not everyone was pleased with the plan. Lieutenant Colonel Michael R. Morgan, the department's chief commissary officer, had formed a dislike of Barton and objected to her tent being placed in proximity to his own.[29] In the end it did not make much difference, for just a week after her arrival General Gillmore ordered Barton off the island, informing her that her services were no longer required there because the sick and wounded soldiers were being forwarded to Beaufort. He directed her to join them there, promising to provide her with "a comfortable dwelling" once she arrived.[30]

Gillmore's order infuriated Barton. She took pride in the sacrifices she had made for the Union, and she viewed the order as critical of her services. As proof of his malicious intentions, Barton claimed the general gave her just "three hours in which to pack, remove, and ship, four tons of supplies with no assistance," even though he knew she had "but one old female negro cook" to assist her. Barton's friends pitched in and helped her meet the deadline, but Gillmore's directive left her bitter and angry. As for aiding the sick and wounded soldiers in Beaufort, she would have none of it. Dorothea Dix's nurses ran the hospitals there, and she had no intention of taking orders from *them*. Instead, Barton returned to Hilton Head, where she fired off a sharp letter to Gillmore complaining of her treatment. The general refused to apologize, however, instead accusing her of putting her ego ahead of the soldiers' welfare. His charge struck a nerve. From that day on, Barton viewed him as her sworn enemy.[31]

Looking back, it's hard to understand Barton's hostile reaction to the order. If the wounded were being sent to the rear, it only made sense that she should join them there. Perhaps Gillmore was right; Barton *was* letting her ego get in the way of duty. She was likely the only woman on Morris Island and, as such, received a great deal of flattering attention from both the medical staff and the soldiers. On the other hand, at Beaufort she would be just one of many female nurses and would not get the attention she craved. But that's only half of the explanation. There was also the matter of subordination. On Morris Island, Barton worked under the general direction of the medical staff but otherwise enjoyed relative liberty. At Beaufort that would not be the case. There, she might have to take orders from other women—women she viewed as not only her inferiors but her rivals. That her pride and vanity would not allow.

Barton had backed herself into a corner. She could not return to the field hospital at Morris Island without Gillmore's consent, and she could not work at Beaufort without losing face. With both options closed, her usefulness in South Carolina was at an end. "My *sympathy* is not destroyed," she asserted in her diary, "but my *confidence* in my ability to accomplish anything of an alleviating character in *this* Dept. is completely annihilated."[32] She continued to furnish supplies to one or two hospitals in the department, and she sent the black residents of St. Helena tons of goods when their island was hit by smallpox, but she did little in the way of nursing.[33] The time had come for her to leave. As the year drew to a close, she packed her bags, distributed what remained of her supplies, and stepped aboard the U.S.S. *Arago* for the long trip home. Behind her she left memories both bitter and sweet. What awaited her, she did not know.[34]

A NEW CAMPAIGN BECKONS

For the next four months Barton was at loose ends. She briefly considered returning to her job at the Patent Office, but she must have known a desk job would no longer satisfy her. "I have nothing to dare or endure in these days," she complained. Ideally, she wished to return to the Army of the Potomac, but as yet she lacked permission to go there. Feeling useless and unappreciated, she slid into depression. Only a return to the army could restore her spirits.[35] That time was fast approaching. In March 1864, President Lincoln promoted Ulysses S. Grant to lieutenant general and appointed him General in Chief of the Armies of the United States. When Barton learned that Grant intended to make his headquarters with the Army of the Potomac, she knew that hard fighting lay ahead and determined to join the army at any cost.

To shield her reputation as a lady while at the front, Barton needed a male protector, someone who could advise her and at the same time provide what she described as "a helping hand and a heart and head ready to act in concert with me." Cornie Welles, Archibald Shaver, and her brother David had filled that role in the past; she hoped that her cousin Leander Poor would fill it now. Poor, then thirty years old, was a graduate of Bowdoin College. Up to this point, he had been serving as a corporal in the United States Engineers, but Barton hoped to have him bumped up to an officer, transferred to the Quartermaster Department, and personally assigned to her. As usual, she turned to Henry Wilson for help. "The coming campaign is to be active[,] sanguinary and final," she wrote to her powerful friend. "I wanted to be in it. I wanted my cousin, whom I could trust implicitly[,] to accompany me, with a rank that would secure me against buffoonery and command such facilities as would effectuate my labor and increase my usefulness." The obliging senator promised to help.[36]

Through Poor, Barton hoped to gain direct access to the army larder. Perhaps he might even use his position to construct a warehouse for her at government expense. Such actions might not be strictly legal, but what of that? Was is not for the good of the soldiers? Apparently Daniel Rucker—now a brigadier general—thought so. After all, in the past had he not loaned her government wagons and teamsters? Still, not everyone was as patriotic as her old friend. There were those, like General Gillmore, who might try to thwart her efforts, either by blocking Leander's appoint-ment or by preventing him from assisting her. Such thoughts preyed on Barton's mind. "I[t] seems impossible for me to go forward all alone," she confided to her diary. "I meet so many and so strong rebuffs to the carrying out of any good purpose which I attempt. I have many fears that Leander if appointed cannot be held to accompany me but will be thrust into the Dept to act legitimately and I be left alone as ever."[37]

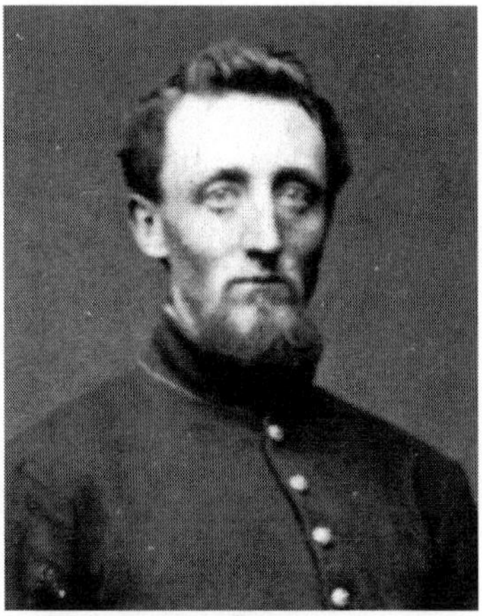

Leander Poor.
(*Library of Congress*)

Uncertainty over Poor's appointment caused Barton to slip back into depression. "Had no courage to get up," she confided to her diary on March 25, "all seemed so dark." Three weeks later she wrote: "Had a most sad down[-]spirited day. All the world appeared selfish and treacherous. I can get no hold on a good noble sentiment any where, and I felt discouraged." When people knocked at her door she did not answer. At times she even flirted with the idea of suicide. "Have been sad all day," she wrote a few days later. "I cannot raise my spirits. the old temptation to go from all the world. I think it will come [to] that some day. it is a struggle for me to keep in society at all. I want to leave all."[38]

News that Wilson had succeeded in getting Poor appointed to the Quartermaster Corps lifted her spirits. Barton immediately determined to pull strings "to secure him to myself," a course of action encouraged by Rucker.[39] The arrival in Washington of the Ninth Corps likewise brightened Barton's mood. After leaving the Army of the Potomac in February 1863, the corps had traveled to Kentucky, Mississippi, and Tennessee. In April 1864, it returned to Virginia as an independent unit assigned to operate in tandem with the Army of the Potomac. As in the summer of 1862, its commander was Maj. Gen. Ambrose E. Burnside.

The Ninth Corps passed through Washington on April 25 and made camp across the Potomac River near Alexandria. Barton wasted no time visiting her old comrades-in-arms. On April 26, she took a steamship across the river and, with the help of a contact in the Quartermaster Corps, secured a wagon and driver to convey her to the camps of the 21st and 57th Massachusetts regiments. She spent the day visiting Dr. Cutter and other friends in the corps before returning to Washington late in the day. The trip buoyed her spirits and made her all the more determined to resume her place in the army. Four days after returning to Washington, she drafted a note to the secretary of war requesting a pass to the front. Until it was approved, all she could do was wait.[40]

As days passed without any action being taken on her pass, Barton again grew despondent. "I was too unhappy and unsettled to write" in my diary, she admitted. "I could get no passes and no one but myself appeared to care or think it was of much consequence."[41] To make matters worse, the armies seemed on the verge of coming to blows. "There are strong rumors of a Battle," she wrote in her diary on May 5. "it is said that our forces have crossed the Rapidan, communication is more than ever obstructed, we hear nothing." The next day only brought more rumors. "The reports are to the effect that the army are in battle, but no one knows." Four days into the campaign and still there was no solid news. "The papers contain little or no intelligence," Barton wrote on May 7. "Every one supposes that the army is in motion, and fighting but no one professes to know. Our Army under Genl. Grant, seems like 'that bourne from whence no traveller returns.'"[42]

Barton got her first reliable intelligence about the fighting from Wilson, who called on her later that day. As chairman of Senate Committee on Military Affairs, he was among the best informed men in Washington, but even his information was sketchy. He confirmed that the Army of the Potomac had engaged the enemy south of the Rapidan River and that the first day's fighting had been successful. But until additional information arrived, that was all he or anyone else in Washington could say.[43] For Barton that was enough. The Army of the Potomac and her beloved Ninth Corps were engaged in battle, and she wanted desperately to join them. For two weeks her application for a pass had been tied up in channels. Direct action was needed. Making out a copy of the application, she handed it to Wilson and asked him to shepherd it through channels. The paper read as follows:

> Washington D.C. April 29/64
> Hon. E. M. Stanton
> Secretary of War—U.S.A.
>
> Sir –
>
> I would most respectfully solicit the favor of your signature to the enclosed, (or a similar form of) Pass permitting me within the lines of our Army.
>
> In requesting this pass I have no intention or desire, to use it unnecessarily, or at an improper time, and I have no object but to aid in relieving the sufferings of our soldiery after battle.
>
> To disabuse your mind of the probable impression that I am some patriotic young lady suddenly seized. with a spirit of adventure, I shall perhaps be pardened [*sic*] a word of explanation. I am not young. A native of Worcester Mass. I have long been a resident of this City. When the "Old Sixth" Mass. Regt. my early school mates were stricken down in Baltimore, Apr 19- 61- I met and cared for them—and from that day to the present, my time, labor[,] strength, thought, and such means as I could command, I have used among our wounded men where they fell.
>
> I have regarded it as a sacred duty. (and I *believe* I have wrought conscientiously). –all the more sacred, that my father was a soldier, following Mad Anthony Wayne through his wild career of war and victory, fighting side by side with Harrison and Johnson, whose friendship he always retained, and when scarce two years ago, feeble and old, he tottered to his grave, he charged me with a dying patriots love to serve and sacrifice for my country in its peril and strengthen and comfort the brave men who stood for its defence. I have tried to obey.
>
> It is possible that I might *never use* the permission that I ask. it would *seem* that the two enormous Commissions, that are driving the charatable [*sic*] world mad of late, must be equal to every contingency. If they only prove as faithful and efficient, as they

> have grown powerful and wealthy we may all rest, quietly, but if the old time cry of wretchednes[s] and suffering without our gates is again to pierce our hearts, I might again wish to reach the scene. Holding your honored pass for such emergency, I will pledge my honor as a lady never to abuse it.
>
> With the highest respect
> I am Most Truly
> Clara Barton
> Washington, D.C.

Appended to the draft of this letter, someone—perhaps Wilson himself—then dictated what the pass should say. The proposed wording would allow Barton to go anywhere at any time and to requisition just about anything from quartermasters.[44]

Wilson took the document, promising to present it to the secretary of war. By the time he did so, the situation in Virginia had become clearer. After crossing the Rapidan River on May 4, Grant had fought Lee to a standstill in a heavily wooded area known as the Wilderness, fifteen miles west of Fredericksburg. Casualties had been staggering: 17,600 Union soldiers and approximately 12,000 Confederates had fallen in just two days of pitched battle. Once again the unhappy town on the Rappahannock River had become, in the words of one soldier, "a city of hospitals."[45] Overwhelmed by the sheer number of casualties, the Army of the Potomac's medical director appealed to Washington for help. The War Department responded by sending an additional 236 surgeons and 775 nurses and medical students to Fredericksburg.[46]

The U.S. Sanitary Commission and the U.S. Christian Commission likewise ramped up their efforts. Both organizations had become active in forwarding supplies to the army since the Battle of Fredericksburg in December 1862. Barton could have joined forces with either commission, but she refused to do so. She viewed both of them with a measure of disdain, considering them to be upstarts and rivals to her own efforts. She had more battlefield experience than delegates of either commission, she believed, and she had no intention of taking orders from them or anybody else. She explained her views to an acquaintance later that month.

> The question would naturally arise with strangers why I, feeling so in unison with the Commissions, among whom I number my dearest friends, should maintain a separate organization. To those who know me, it is obvious. Long before either Commission was in the field, or even had an existence, I was laboring by myself, for the little I might be able to accomplish, & gathering such helpers about me as I was best able to do, and toiling in the front of our armies wherever I could reach, and thus I have labored on, up to the present time. Death has laid his hand upon the active forms of my co-workers, and stilled the steps [of those] most useful to me, but others have arisen to supply the place;—and now, after all this lapse of time, it does not seem wise or desirable to change my course. If, by practice, I have acquired any skill, it belongs to me to use discretionary, and I might not work as efficiently, or labor as happily, under the direction of those of less experience than myself.[47]

One of the coworkers stilled by death was Cornelius Welles. The Baptist missionary was an irrepressible traveler. In August 1863, while Barton was in South Carolina, he had decided to go west. He booked passage on a ship to California and, once there, started overland to Arizona. While passing through Los Angeles County, he fell ill with a coronary ailment. Four days later he was dead.[48] Barton bespoke his praise in a letter to a mutual acquaintance.

> When Cornie Wells died, you lost a friend, and I lost one, and the poor lost a helper, and the sufferer a sympathizer, the sick a healer, the Christian a brother, the sinner *more* than a brother, and the world lost a meek, patient, faithful follower of him who died on Cavalry [*sic*]. . . .
>
> How calmly he spoke, while others shouted in confusion, how steadily he wrought while others stood aghast, how firm he remained where whole columns wavered and how boldly he pressed forward when others fled. These traits proclaim him the brave as well as the true man, and it is meet that I speak of them for to none other can they be known so well. These were characteristics which his friends, who had witnessed only his gentleness in peaceful Christian life might well have doubted, but

> which I, who have seen him face death calmly, bravely and cheerfully, not for the minute, or the hour, but for whole days and nights have learned and honored.[49]

A Washington newspaper recounted Welles's heroic service with Barton at Antietam and Fredericksburg, where the two had rescued the wounded from the field, bound their wounds, and saved them from certain death. It claimed to "have in our possession two of the murderous shells which fell within their tent while thus serving God and their country on the battle-field."[50] And yet in later years, when Barton spoke to audiences about her Civil War experiences, she never once mentioned Welles nor any of her other associates. To do so might have detracted from her own accomplishments, and that would simply not do. Clara Barton craved the spotlight, and she would not share it with anyone—not even Cornie Welles.

5

Return to Fredericksburg

"THAT CITY OF SUFFERING AND DEATH"

BELLE PLAIN

For two days Barton waited to hear about her pass. But by May 10, 1864, her patience had run out. Still having not heard from Henry Wilson, she decided to go to the War Department to look into the matter herself. She got nowhere. She then proceeded to Daniel Rucker's office and, perhaps at his suggestion, decided to apply directly to Surgeon General Joseph Barnes. The doctor refused her "roughly," Barton recalled. Still she would not give up. She had made up her mind to go to Virginia, and go she would. Returning to her apartment, she dashed off a note to Senator Wilson, anxiously inquiring about his success in securing her a pass from the secretary of war.[1]

On May 11, while awaiting Wilson's reply, Barton went to see Gardiner Tufts, head of the Washington office of the Massachusetts state relief agency, a state-sponsored organization that provided for the needs of the Bay State's sick and wounded soldiers.[2] She had been successful in securing the promotion of her cousin Leander Poor, but instead of assigning him to assist her in Virginia the War Department had sent him west to serve with the Army of the Cumberland. Barton felt it improper to travel alone to the army, and she hoped that Tufts might accompany her to Fredericksburg in Poor's place. To her chagrin, she found that he had decided not to go to the front—at least not yet. Meanwhile, thousands of wounded soldiers began pouring into the nation's capital. With no pass and no one to accompany her, Barton gave up all thought of going to the front. No sooner had she abandoned that hope, however, than a special messenger arrived from Rucker bearing the pass that she had fought so hard to get. At the same time, she learned that her acquaintance, J. W. Doe, was preparing to travel to Fredericksburg. As if by Providence, both obstacles to her trip had vanished.[3]

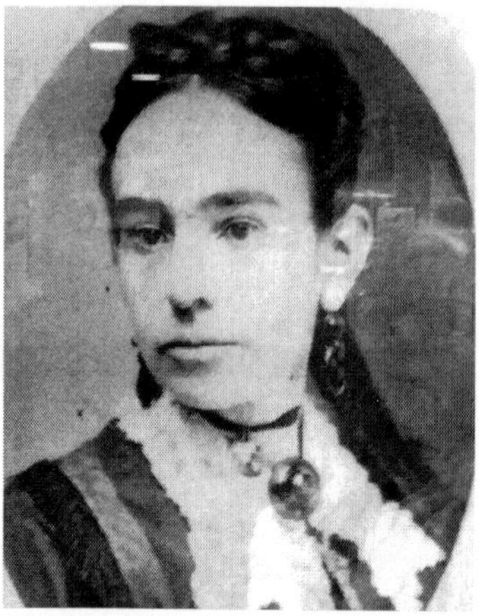
Julia S. Wheelock. (*Kalamazoo College*)

With pass in hand, Barton hurried down to the Seventh Street Wharf and secured passage aboard the steamship *Winona*, which was leaving that afternoon for Belle Plain, the Army of the Potomac's new supply base on Potomac Creek, ten miles east of Fredericksburg. The ship did not leave until four o'clock. In the meantime, she returned to her apartment, dashed off a few letters, and threw together some things for the trip. When she returned to the wharf, she found Rucker there. She undoubtedly thanked him for getting her a pass and may have asked him for an order that would enable her to requisition transportation and supplies from the Quartermaster Department once she reached Fredericksburg.[4]

The *Winona* cast off its lines late that afternoon. On board was an infantry regiment, a battery of artillery, and dozens of relief workers, including Elmina Brainerd and Julia S. Wheelock of the Michigan Soldiers' Relief Association and William Howell Reed of the U.S. Christian Commission. Just a few miles downriver, the *Winona* was involved in a collision and had to tie up for repairs at Alexandria. It remained there overnight and continued its journey the next day. As the ship plied its way south down the Potomac River a cold front swept through, lashing the region with heavy rains.[5]

The *Winona* reached Belle Plain at 1 P.M. on May 12. Reed viewed the improvised supply base as it came into sight. "A simple beach, with richly-wooded hills, rose abruptly from the water, from which long piers, hastily extemporized out of pontoon boats ran out into the river. . . . All seemed to be in inextricable confusion. In the river were barges, steamers, propellers, and transports—some at anchor, some discharging, some arriving, some departing, and all jammed together in confusion . . . while on shore were tired mules and broken-down horses, army wagons and ambulances, stuck hopelessly in the mud." To Reed, it appeared to be "a surging, concentrated mass of intense activity and suffering."[6]

The *Winona* anchored offshore awaiting permission to dock, taking its place among seventy-five other steamers and transports that were waiting to discharge their passengers and cargo.[7] In less than a week's time, the Union army had transformed the quiet landing into one of the busiest ports in all America. Supplies were taken by ship down the Potomac River, unloaded at Belle Plain, and carried by wagon to the front. Surgeons then placed wounded soldiers aboard the empty wagons for the trip back. Many stopped for care at improvised hospitals in Fredericksburg. The rest went directly to Belle Plain, there to be placed aboard ships and transported to general hospitals in the North.

The road between Fredericksburg and Belle Plain wound through ten miles of bleak countryside rendered treeless by the army's encampment there two years earlier. Bands of Confederate guerrillas boldly roamed the area, attacking any wagons that ventured forth without a proper guard. As it neared Potomac Creek, the road passed through a narrow defile and descended to the landing, which was located on a broad patch of clay adjacent to the river.[8] Federal forces had occupied Belle Plain just a few days earlier, and the wharf was in wretched condition. On the day that Barton arrived the structure gave way, delaying embarkation of the wounded for nearly twelve hours. A team of five hundred engineers hurried to the landing to make the necessary repairs, but it was clear that if the Union army was going to remain in the area for an extended period of time, it would need a better base of supply.[9]

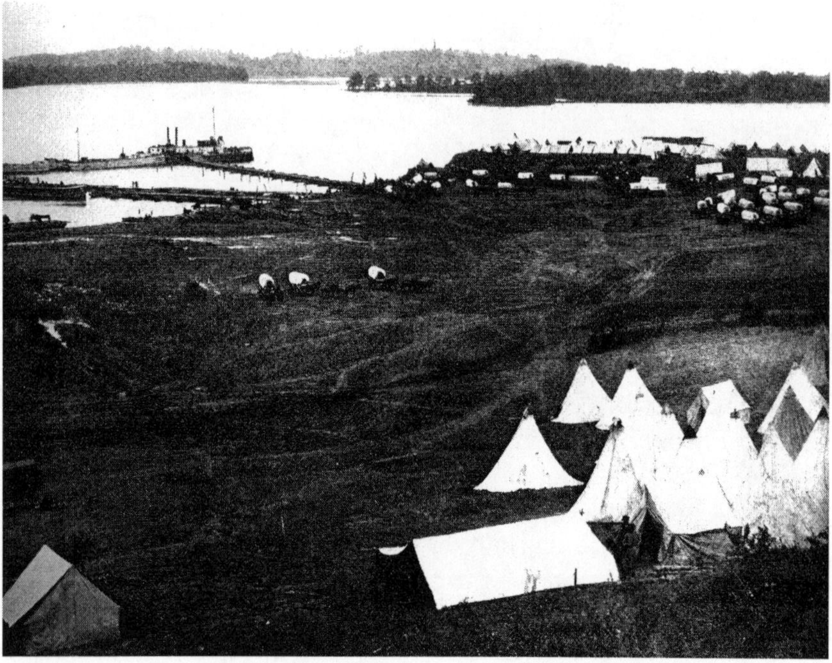

Belle Plain. (*Francis T. Miller*, Photographic History of the Civil War)

While work crews struggled to repair the wharf, the Army of the Potomac engaged Lee's Confederates in battle twenty miles away at Spotsylvania Court House. Unable to land, the *Winona*'s passengers gathered in the ship's cabin to pray. Barton joined them. "The meeting was a most solemn and impressive one," remembered Julia Wheelock. "The afternoon was dark and gloomy, the sky overcast with clouds, and the rain falling; while ever and anon our ears were saluted with the boom of the cannon, which plainly indicated that the conflict was still raging, and every moment new names were added to the long list of sufferers. The solemnity of the occasion, and the deep impressions then made, must—it seems to me—follow each of us through life."[10]

At sunset, Barton and the other passengers transferred from the *Winona* to a lighter-draft vessel called *Young America*, which carried them to the landing.[11] It was still pouring outside, however, and the passengers wisely decided to remain on board ship until the next day.

It was 9 A.M., May 13, before they finally went ashore.[12] "I shall never forget the scene which met my eye as I stepped from the Boat to the top of the ridge," Barton wrote. "Standing in this plain of mortar mud were at least 200 six-mule army wagons, crowded full of wounded men waiting to be taken upon the boats for Washington. They had driven from Fredericksburg that morning. Each driver had gotten his wagon as far as he could, for those in front of and about him had stopped. Of the depth of the mud the best judgment was formed from the fact that no entire hub of a wheel was in sight and you saw nothing of any animal below its knees and the mass of mud all settled into place perfectly smooth and glassy."[13] She later described the landing as a "10 acre mortar bed."[14]

The relief workers immediately sprang into action, wading through the knee-deep mud to deliver crackers, coffee, and bread to the half-starved soldiers lying in the ambulances.[15] Barton joined the effort. In company with Elmina Brainerd, she trudged up the hillside to a U.S. Christian Commission tent run by thirty-five-year-old James Cruikshanks, a Congregationalist minister born in Scotland but was now residing in Spencer, Massachusetts.[16] As Barton gazed upon the busy scene before her, a young minister serving with the Commission—possibly Cruikshanks himself—lamented their inability to help the wounded men waiting in the ambulances below. Barton replied that there *was* something they could do: they could feed them. "For a moment," Barton recalled, "his countenance brightened then fell again as quickly as he exclaimed: '*What a pity*! We have a great deal of clothing and reading matter, but no food in any quantity excepting crackers.' I replied that I had coffee and that between us I thought we could arrange to give them all hot coffee and crackers. 'But where shall we make our coffee?' he asked as he gazed wistfully about the bare, wet hillside. I pointed to a little hollow beside a stump and said, 'There was a good place for a fire and any of this loose brush will do.'"

In a matter of minutes, the two had a dozen kettles of hot coffee simmering over an open fire. The minister cheered but only briefly. Soon his face again bore a troubled aspect. "Our crackers are in barrels, and we have neither basket nor box. How can we carry them?" he asked. "Aprons would be better than either," replied his more experienced companion, "and getting something as near the size and shape of a common table-cloth as I could find, tied one about each of us, fastening all four of the corners to the waist and pinned the sides, thus leaving one hand for a kettle of coffee and one free to administer it."

The two tramped down the hillside. When they reached the bottom, they encountered a sea of mud. Barton's hapless companion again became despondent. "How are we to get to them?" he asked. "There is no way but to walk to them," Barton replied. With that, she strode into the mire, her associate following timidly in her wake. "I found myself striving hard to keep the muscles of my face all straight," she later told audiences, "and the corners of my mouth would draw into wickedness as with a backward glance I saw the good man tighten his grasp upon his apron and take his first step in military life."[17] The incident made two points important to Barton: it underscored her own toughness and, just as important, it demonstrated her superiority to the timorous and inexperienced delegates of the U.S. Christian Commission.

Among the soldiers encountered by Barton as she helped distribute the food was Capt. Thomas R. Keenan of the 56th Massachusetts. Although he had been shot in the neck, Keenan managed to tell Barton that the 59th regiment's commander, Col. Jacob P. Gould, was suffering from sunstroke and that division commander Brig. Gen. Thomas G. Stevenson had been killed by a stray rebel bullet.[18] Gould would recover only to suffer a fatal wound at the Battle of the Crater ten weeks later.

ONE VAST HOSPITAL

Barton spent that night in a tent, the rain drumming against her canvas roof.[19] For two days it had come down, and still it showed no signs of stopping. The area roads, bad enough under ordinary conditions, became muddy quagmires. Fortunately, Barton and Brainerd were able to secure a ride into town with a lieutenant named Carr. On the way they passed seven thousand Confederate prisoners, who had been captured in the fighting at Spotsylvania.[20] The women reached Fredericksburg about noon on May 14, one day after William Howell Reed.[21] The U.S. Sanitary Commission delegate

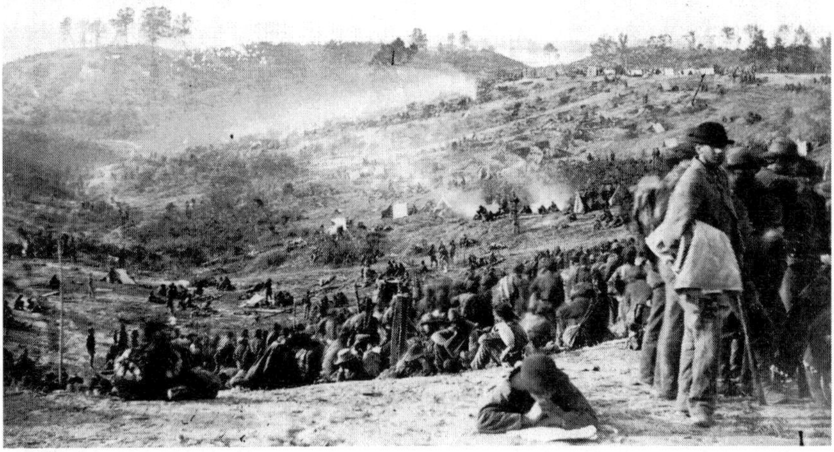

Confederate prisoners at Belle Plain. (*Library of Congress*)

thought that "the crumbling town, deserted by its population, ruined by the conflicts which had twice raged through its streets, gave it an appearance of death, from which it seemed that there could be no resurrection." Wounded soldiers packed the streets from end to end. More than twenty-six thousand sick and wounded men would pass through it that month, five times its antebellum population. "Fredericksburg is one vast Hospital," wrote a Sixth Corps staff officer. "The 'red flag' & wounded men appear everywhere."[22]

The Medical Department struggled to cope with the enormous influx of patients. A New Hampshire state relief agent, who reached the town the same day as Barton, reported, "In Fredericksburg I found a want of nearly all kinds of stores [and] owing to the bad roads and the urgent demand for supplies at the front, it was impossible for a few days for Fredericksburg to receive a sufficient quantity. The great need was for straw and hay for the men to lie upon: many had but a blanket and others not that[,] and every house seemed thus occupied."[23]

Julia Wheelock found a shortage of food as well as bedding. "Such scenes of wretchedness and of terrible suffering I have never before witnessed," she wrote. "I found the wounded lying upon the hard floor without pillows, and many without a blanket, so closely crowded together that there was scarcely room to pass between them. Officers and soldiers are lying side by side. . . . To the untold suffering experienced from broken bones and shattered limbs, is added that of hunger, many having eaten nothing for three and four days previous to their arrival here; and thus they are dying not only of wounds, but of starvation."[24] Barton found the same thing among soldiers lying on the sides of the streets. "They had been wounded two and three days previous," she wrote, "had been bro[ugh]t from the front, and after all this lay still another night without care or food, or shelter, many doubtless famished after arriving in Fredericksburg."[25]

More pressing even than the need for food was the demand for trained medical personnel. When the army first occupied Fredericksburg on May 9 it brought just thirty surgeons. As wounded men began pouring into the city, the Medical Department sent a plea to Washington asking for assistance. The surgeon general replied by rushing surgeons, nurses, and medical students to Fredericksburg; however, most of them had not yet reached the town. "A few of the glorious Sanitary had reached," wrote Barton, "but what could they do among so many[?] A few noble volunteer surgeons had reached, and Oh how they tried but the work grew upon their hands & what could they do[?]"[26]

Had the Rappahannock River been open to shipping as far upriver as Fredericksburg or had the railroad been in operation to Aquia Landing, surgeons could have alleviated the congestion in town. But they were not. Corduroy roads between Fredericksburg and Belle Plain provided the only means by which the army could evacuate soldiers to Washington, and the jolting ride was too rough for most of the wounded men to bear. Consequently the town became a deadly bottleneck.[27] "Only those most slightly wounded have been taken on to W[ashington]," wrote Barton in despair. "the roads are fearful, and it is worth the life of a wounded man to move him over them. . . . A common ambulance is scarce sufficient to get through. We passed them this morning four miles out of town full of wounded with the tangs broken or wheels crushed in the middle of a hill, in

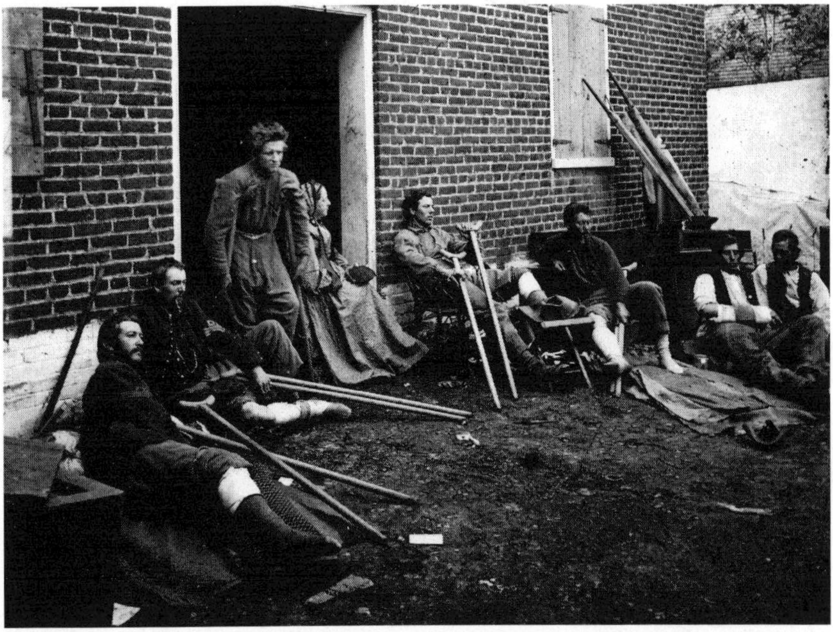

Wounded Union soldiers at Fredericksburg, May 1864. (*Library of Congress*)

mud from one to two feet deep. what was to be done with the moaning suffering occupants God only knew."[28]

The Medical Department was in a fix. If it sent patients to Belle Plain over the wretched roads, they would surely die; if it kept them in Fredericksburg, they would just as surely starve. "Dr. Hitchcock most strongly and earnestly and *indignantly* remonstrates against any more removals of broken or amputated limbs," Barton reported. "He declares it little better than murder, and says the greater proportion of them will die there, if not better fed and afforded more room, and better air. The surgeons do *all* they *can* but no provisions have been made for such a wholesale slaughter on the part of anyone, and I believe it would be impossible to comprehend the magnitude of the necessity without witnessing it."[29]

For the next twenty hours Barton witnessed suffering on an unimaginable scale. Upon arriving in Fredericksburg, she accompanied Elmina Brainerd to the headquarters of the Michigan Soldiers' Relief Association, where she encountered Pvt. James Barker, an acquaintance from Worcester who was serving in the 15th Massachusetts. Barker knew his way around town, and at Barton's request he led her to the Methodist Episcopal Church (South), which was being used as a hospital by the Ninth Corps's First Division, the one previously commanded by Samuel Sturgis. There, at the southwest corner of George and Charles Streets, she found eight officers and dozens of men of the 57th Massachusetts stretched out on blankets across the floor. The regiment had incurred heavy casualties in the campaign and was down to just two hundred men.[30]

Corporal Josiah B. Hall was among those wounded in the Wilderness one week earlier. Barton's cousin Lt. George E. Barton had been in charge of the ambulance train that had brought him to Fredericksburg. "As soon as I was made as comfortable as possible on the floor of the Southern M. E. Church," remembered Hall, "Captain [*sic*] Barton found Miss Barton, told her where I was and that I was thought to be mortally wounded. My exhausted condition at that time was such that I have only an indistinct recollection of the first aid Miss Barton gave me, but later when my father, who was with the Sanitary Commission arrived, I had many evidences of her watchful care of me." Clara Barton had Hall taken out of the crowded building and moved into a private house, where he remained until she found him transportation to the North.[31]

While at the church, Barton met a member of the U.S. Christian Commission, who escorted her to Planter's Hotel, a large building located at the northwest corner of William Street and Charles. Surgeons had converted the building into a hospital for Brig. Gen. Orlando B. Willcox's division of the Ninth Corps, and it was packed "from ground to garret" with four hundred wounded soldiers, "not one in ten of whom," Barton noted, "could rise and stand." Most of the men belonged to Western regiments.[32] "I was struck with their fine soldierly figures and features remarkable even in terrible extremity," she wrote, "and stopping by one I asked 'where are you from—' 'Michigan,' and so on 'Michigan,' 'Michigan,' up one flight of stairs and another. Still 'Michigan.' At length in my surprise I said without reflection, 'Did Michigan take up this hand and play it alone?' 'Yes,' faintly answered a poor fellow at my feet . . . , 'Yes, and got Euchered.' I thought he was correct."[33]

Like the patients in the First Division hospital, Wilcox's men suffered from a lack of attention and supplies. None of them had cots nor even straw to lie upon. Even the worst cases had to stretch out on the hard wooden floors. Worse still, most had received no medical attention whatsoever. "A great number of them were to undergo amputation sometime," Barton noted in her diary, "but no surgeons yet. They had not clippers [surgeons] for one in ten. I saw no stove in any hospital, and no mattresses." Disease compounded the soldiers' distress. Gangrene had infected many of the wounds, and erysipelas, an inflammation of the skin caused by viral infection, had begun to spread throughout the wards.[34]

The most immediate danger, however, was malnutrition. The men had had nothing to eat all day and were weak with hunger. Barton had a basket of hardtack left over from the previous day, and she proceeded to give each man half a cracker and a sip of coffee until her meager supply ran out. It angered her that she did not have more to give. "My heart sickens," she wrote her friend Frances D. Gage later in the week. "Such streets full of dying men, such trains of wounded, such packed churches and old hotels, crowded with agony; and worse than all, the faint 'Nothing' always echoed to your inquiry, 'What have you to eat? Are you very hungry?' 'Oh! so hungry and so faint.' I looked on, and broke crackers in two, to feed out to starving men, till it came to be a reproach to me that I was there, instead of being elsewhere gathering up supplies." Then and there she made up her mind to return to Washington for additional food.[35]

Barton rose early on Sunday, May 15, and hurried from her lodging at the U.S. Christian Commission headquarters to the provost marshal's office, where she had taken supper the night before.[36] For the fifth straight day the rain continued to fall. Hundreds of wagons crowded the muddy streets, their pallets packed with wounded soldiers, many in the final throes of death. "Many died in the wagons," remembered Barton, "and their companions, where they had sufficient strength[,] had raised up and thrown them out into the street. I saw them lying there early this morning. They had been wounded two and three days previous, had been bro[ugh]t from the front, and after all this lay still another night without care or food or shelter, many doubtless famished after arriving in Fredericksburg."[37]

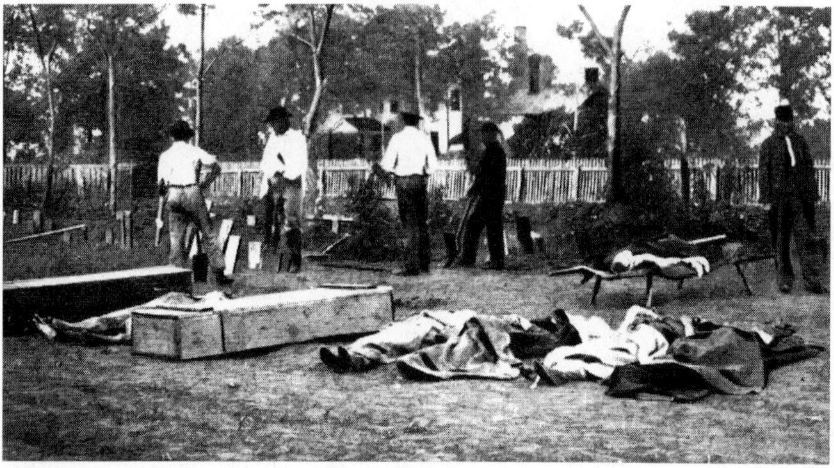

Corpses awaiting burial, Fredericksburg 1864. (*Francis T. Miller*, Photographic History of the Civil War)

Barton blamed the soldiers' deaths on city residents who refused to admit the wounded men into their homes. Even more culpable, she felt, were Union officers in charge of the town who refused to make them do so.[38] "No person present has forgotten the heart sickness which spread over the entire country as the busy wires flashed the dire tidings of the terrible destitution and suffering of these same wounded of the wilderness to whom I have alluded as they lay in Fredericksburg," she later told her audiences. "But you may never have known how many hundred fold those ills were augmented by the unfortunate detail of improper, heartless, unfaithful officers to the immediate command of the city upon whose action and decisions depended entirely the *care, shelter, food, comfort* and *lives* of that whole city of wounded men. One of the highest officers I found there is since a convicted traitor," she asserted. "And another little dapper Captain of 21, quartered with the owners of one of the finest mansions in the town, boasted that he had changed his opinion since entering the city in his present capacity the day before. 'That it *was*, in fact, a pretty hard thing for refined people like the citizens of Fredericksburg, to be compelled to open their houses and admit these dirty, lousy, common soldiers *and he was not going to compel it.*'"[39]

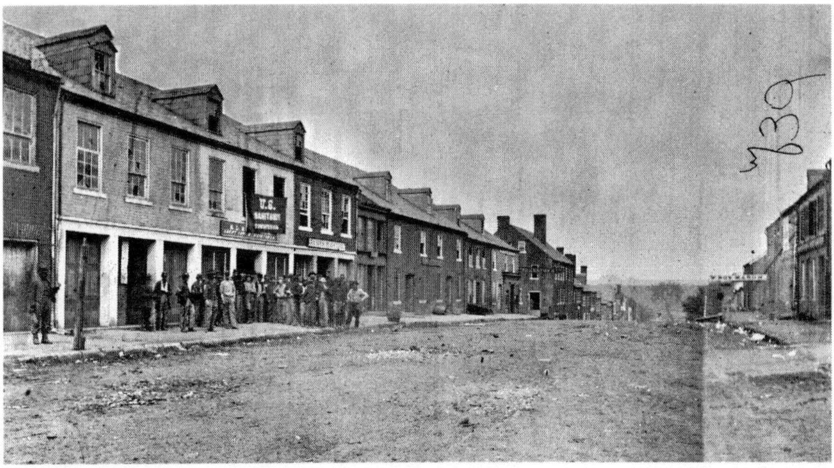

Fredericksburg in May 1864. (*Library of Congress*)

The officer's declaration made Barton's blood boil. Although she had been in Fredericksburg less than a day, she had seen enough to convince her that the officers in charge there were grossly incompetent, if not traitorous, and that scores of wounded men were perishing each day as a result. This conviction sharpened her desire to return to Washington as soon as possible. "I remember[ed] one man there who would set it right, if he knew it; who possessed the power and who would believe me if I told him," she wrote.[40] That man was Henry Wilson.

BACK IN WASHINGTON

Barton wasted no time executing her plan. Hurrying across town, she entered the provost marshal's office and insisted on "immediate conveyance back to Belle Plain."[41] It was a brazen demand, given the tremendous need for ambulances at that time, and the officer in charge properly refused to comply. Instead, he sent her to see Col. Edmund Schriver, who was in command of the town. He in turn directed her to Capt. James E. Jones, the assistant quartermaster in charge of ground transportation at Belle Plain, who must have had an office in Fredericksburg. Jones acceded to Barton's demands, providing her with an ambulance drawn by four stout horses, which she shortly exchanged for a light army wagon. With her, as an escort, went Henry A. Goodrich, a prominent merchant from Fitchburg, Massachusetts, and treasurer of the town's Bounty Fund.[42]

Barton later told audiences that she rode "ten miles at an unbroken gallop thro' field and swamp and stumps and mud to Belle Plain" on her mission of mercy, but like many so of her later assertions, that is a gross exaggeration.[43] Horses cannot maintain a gallop for such a distance and certainly not while pulling a wagon. Given the execrable condition of the roads, it is lucky she reached her destination at all. As it was, the team brought Barton and Goodrich to Belle Plain at 2 p.m., covering the eight-mile distance in approximately six hours. Barton immediately applied for transportation to Washington. Capt. Perley S. Pitkin, the assistant quartermaster in charge of transports, secured her and Goodrich passage aboard the *Silver Star*, a steam tug that was just about to pull away from the dock. As Barton was about to board, she ran into Colonel Gould, who was himself awaiting transportation to Washington. She exchanged a few hasty words with the colonel and furnished him with a brush and some soap. In return, he gave her five dollars to aid the troops.[44]

The *Silver Star* reached Alexandria at six o'clock that evening. There Barton caught another ship that took her across the Potomac River to Washington. By 7 P.M. she was back in the nation's capital. Despite the lateness of the hour, she sent a message to Wilson asking him to meet her at once. He arrived within the hour, whereupon Barton told him about the "suffering and faithlessness" in Fredericksburg. Goodrich probably confirmed her story. As further proof, she carried written statements by Dr. Hitchcock and Captain Jones testifying to the horrid conditions in the town. Shocked by these revelations, Wilson started for the War Department with Barton in tow. Although it was then 10 P.M., the powerful senator demanded and received an immediate audience with Secretary of War Edwin M. Stanton.[45]

The secretary undoubtedly resented the late-night intrusion, and Barton found him "not quite affable." He listened impatiently as Wilson repeated Barton's charges of mismanagement by Fredericksburg's military authorities. Stanton was skeptical of the report. According to Barton, he felt that Wilson "must have been

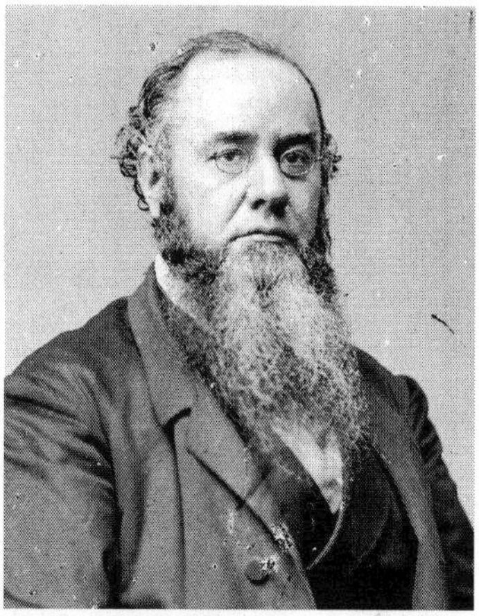

Secretary of War Edwin M. Stanton (*Library of Congress*)

deceived by some frightened civilian" as he had received no reports of unusual suffering at the town and military authorities had sought no special assistance. Wilson assured him that "the officers in trust there were not to be relied upon. They were faithless, overcome by the blandishments of the wily inhabitants." When Stanton still hesitated to act, Wilson issued an ultimatum. "One of two things will be done," he threatened. "Either you will send some-one to-night with authority to investigate and correct the abuses of our wounded men at Fredericksburg, or the Senate will send someone tomorrow."[46] Stanton knew when he was licked. That night, he wrote out an order for Quartermaster General Montgomery Meigs to proceed at once to Fredericksburg, evaluate the situation, and make any changes he deemed necessary.[47]

After that, action came quickly. "At 2 o'clock in the morning, the Qt. Master Gen'l and Staff galloped to the Sixth Street wharf under orders," Barton triumphantly told her listeners. "At *10* they were in Fredericksburg. At *noon*, the wounded were fed from the food of the city, and the houses were opened to the *dirty, lousy soldiers* of the Union Army. Both railroad and canal were opened. In three days, I returned with carloads of supplies. No more jolting in army-wagons. And every man who left Fredericksburg by boat or car owes it to the firm decision of one man that his grating bones were not dragged 10 miles across the country or left to Bleach in the sands of that traitorous city."[48] One man and, by inference, one woman: Clara Barton.

As usual, however, Barton's claims outdistanced her actual accomplishments. Her trip to Washington, while it may have prompted Secretary of War Stanton to dispatch Meigs to Fredericksburg, did not result in any major changes in the care of the wounded there for the simple reason that none were needed. By May

17, Medical Department officials, led by Surgeon Edward B. Dalton, had matters well in hand—or at least as much as conditions would allow. Upon arriving in the town, Dalton reported taking possession of the "churches, public buildings, warehouses, mills, and the more commodious of the private dwellings . . . for hospital purposes," adding that "a large number of wounded officers and men were billeted upon such families as still remained in town."[49]

Private accounts back up his statement. A correspondent for the *New York Evening Post* writing from Fredericksburg on May 14, the day Barton arrived in Fredericksburg, confirmed that "almost every house is to-day a hospital; the churches are crowded with wounded and dying soldiers. . . . The stores and warehouses are filled with sick and suffering ones. . . . You walk in the cool of the evening along the streets, and at every window you see a bandaged face. At many doors, if you have courage to look you will see groups of surgeons around little tables cutting, sawing, and chatting and laughing the while." Four days later Deloss Burton, a soldier in the 50th New York Engineers, wrote that "Every church, hotel, store, shop, house, store house, is crowded with wounded." A civilian concurred, writing that "Every house, barn, and shed is a hospital." There *was* a housing shortage in Fredericksburg that May, but it was because there were so many patients, not because the buildings were not being used.[50]

Barton likewise overstated her impact in opening the Richmond, Fredericksburg, and Potomac Railroad. Confederate forces had damaged the railroad between Fredericksburg and Aquia Landing one year earlier. At first, that was not important because Grant's lines of supply and communication ran through Brandy Station rather than Fredericksburg. However, as Grant pushed south toward Spotsylvania Court House he cut his connections with Brandy Station and opened a new line of supply with Washington via the Potomac River. At that point, he would have found the railroad quite useful. But Grant realized that rebuilding the R. F. & P. Railroad between Fredericksburg and Aquia Landing would take at least a week, and he did not expect to be in the area that long. Rather than reconstructing the railroad, he ordered the Quarter-master Department to establish a temporary supply base at Belle Plain.

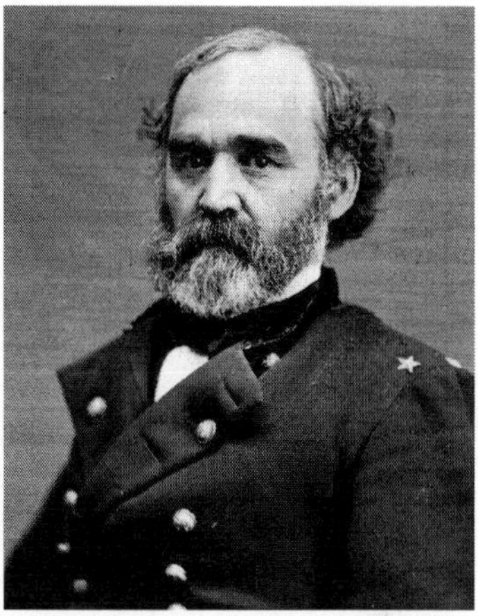

Quartermaster General Montgomery Meigs. (*Library of Congress*)

Stubborn resistance by Lee's army altered his plans. After a week of heavy fighting, the Union commander found himself bogged down in front of Spotsylvania Court House with prolonged rains forcing the general to temporarily suspend military operations. Meanwhile, thousands of wounded soldiers collected at Fredericksburg awaiting transportation to the rear. Confronted with this crisis, Union authorities began inspecting the railroad on May 14 to determine how long it would take to put it into operation. They finished their examination two days later. On May 16, Chief of Staff Henry Halleck notified Grant that the railroad could be repaired in eight days and asked if it should be done. That same day, the Army of the Potomac's commander, George G. Meade, notified Grant that six thousand wounded men had arrived in Fredericksburg and recommended that the railroad be rebuilt. Grant concurred. On May 17, he sent a dispatch to Halleck ordering him to repair the railroad at once.[51] Meigs had arrived in Fredericksburg the previous morning in time to report on this development and perhaps facilitate it, but he did not initiate it.[52]

If Barton's late-night meeting with Stanton did not have any impact in alleviating the housing and transportation problems in Fredericksburg, it may have had some role in increasing the flow of supplies there. Representatives of the Citizens Committee of Fitchburg, Massachusetts, noted that "about the 17th or 18th inst. new vigor was evinced, and vastly more ample supplies arrived at Belle Plain, with the needed wagons and horses for transit to Fredericksburg, both from the Government proper and from the two Commissions. When we left, on the 21st inst., there was no longer a destitution."[53] Even then, the importance of Barton's role is open to question. The Fitchburg commissioners' comment that the much-needed supplies came not only from the government but also from the Christian and Sanitary Commissions suggests that others beside Barton were responding to the crisis.

While all this was going on, Barton remained in Washington amassing supplies for the army. She got to bed well after midnight after her meeting with Stanton and Wilson and awoke on May 16 feeling hungry and faint. She restored her strength with not one, but two, hearty meals before heading to the Quartermaster Department to line up food and transportation for her return to Fredericksburg. Rucker promised to give her the necessary transportation, but she would need special authorization to procure commissary supplies. For that, she would have to go to Wilson. Barton sat down at once and wrote her powerful friend a statement about the dire conditions that she had found in Fredericksburg, ending her letter with a request for supplies. With the letter she enclosed a similar statement by her colleague Henry Goodrich. She sent copies of the documents both to Wilson and to his senatorial colleague, Charles Sumner.[54]

Meanwhile, word of Barton's activities was spreading to the outside world. While in Washington, Goodrich ran into a correspondent for the *Fitchburg Sentinel*. Goodrich told the reporter about the horrid conditions in Fredericksburg and how his delegation was trying to ameliorate the suffering. He then went on to describe the mission that had brought him and Barton back to Washington. Impressed by what Goodrich told him, the reporter included a glowing tribute to Barton in his next column.

> Miss Clara Barton, of Worcester, who has been on nearly every battle-field in which the "Army of the Potomac" has been engaged, *doing and daring* as few women ever did, or can, is, as usual, in the midst of the suffering and dying at the front, looking after our Worcester county boys, but extending her care and sympathies to all. She has very appropriately been classed among the "Florence Nightingales" of America, whose heroism and patriotism has entitled them to this distinguished name—and yet I venture the assertion that no one has ever "stood their ground" amid shot and shell and kept on in their work of mercy, at the im[m]inent risk of limb and life, in as many exposed points, as

> Miss Barton. Yet heaven has kindly protected a[nd] preserved her; and, were it proper for me to present the facts as they exist, and to say what she is doing to remedy existing disabilities, you would give her the highest mead of praise, gratitude, and respect. Suffice it to say, that she has hastily returned here to communicate with high officials, on matters connected with the comfort and welfare of our sick and wounded.[55]

It would take time for those "high officials" to respond. In the meantime, Barton returned to her apartment to rest. She was then forty-two years old, and the long hours of toil were beginning to take their toll. An acquaintance dropped by to see her, but she pushed him out the door as soon as possible and then threw herself down on the couch. Within minutes she was asleep. When she awoke, it was midnight. Undressing, she retired for the night and slept for another twelve hours.[56]

The sun was climbing toward its zenith when Barton arose on May 17. After fortifying herself with a hearty breakfast, she headed across town to talk with Gardiner Tufts, chairman of the Massachusetts state relief agency. She asked Tufts to speak with Wilson in regard to procuring government supplies for her to take to Fredericksburg. Tufts collared Wilson later in the day but was unsuccessful. Apparently, even a senator could not properly allocate government supplies to a private individual, no matter how good her intentions might be. Wilson broke the news to Barton himself that evening. While he could not grant her request for supplies, he did promise to secure her a pass back to the front.[57]

There was little point in returning to Fredericksburg if she had nothing to give the wounded soldiers, though. She needed supplies and lots of them. But where to find them? She had exhausted all of the supplies in her possession, and many of the groups that had supported her earlier in the war were now sending their contributions to the Sanitary Commission, the Christian Commission, or one of the many state relief agencies. And even if she succeeded in accumulating a large supply of goods, where would she store them and who would safeguard them while she was at the front?

On May 18, she went to the Treasury Department to discuss the matter with an old friend, the Reverend William M. Ferguson. Barton proposed issuing a nationwide appeal for supplies if Ferguson would store them for her in his office inside the Treasury Building. Ferguson agreed, whereupon Barton sat down at his desk and drafted the following plea to the people of the North.[58]

> To the Clergy and Soldiers' Friends:
> WASHINGTON, May 16th, 1864.
>
> BRETHREN AND FRIENDS:—For the first time in the history of the war, the magnitude and intensity of suffering and want are so appalling as to wring from me a public call for aid.
>
> I have just returned from Fredericksburg, where I have used and sent my last pound of supplies. Would it be pardonable if I ask you to aid in filling my hands that I may help meet the distress crowded within the dingy streets of that city of suffering and death. I will not pain you with description. The published accounts, although carefully given, are sufficient to point the necessity. All there are doing what they can, and still the suffering continues and the battles rage. There is time for all to labor and grow weary in well doing.
>
> I beg you to forward what you can collect, without delay, of food suitable for wounded men, or the means to purchase it.
>
> Yours, very truly,
> CLARA BARTON.
>
> Please send to address of Rev. Wm. Ferguson, Treasurer's Office, U.S. Treasury, Washington, D.C., for CLARA BARTON.[59]

Barton dated her appeal May 16, but her diary makes it clear that she actually drafted it two days later.[60] It was the first and only time during the war that she publicly asked for help. Frances Gage urged the public to support her friend's efforts. In a letter to the *National Anti-Slavery Standard* in June 1864, Gage wrote: "Clara Barton! Oh! if others, if all people knew her as I know her, that call would fill her hands, and with her hands full, no suffering that could be relieved by mortals would long be abated. No woman, perhaps, in the Union has done more than Miss B. on the battle-fields and in the front since the war began, and yet so modest is she that few except those who have come into personal contact with her know her worth and reliability. I hope she will be generously aided."[61]

Among those who responded to Barton's call was Mrs. D. C. Alling of New York. When later writing to Alling to thank her for her donation, Barton explained what had prompted the nationwide appeal. "I have been always able to meet my own demands, with such supplies as came voluntarily from my circle of personal friends, which fortunately was not small. But the necessities of the present campaign were well nigh overwhelming, and my duty required that I gather all I could, even if I shouted aloud to strangers, for those who lay fainting and speechless by the way-side, or moaning in the Wilderness. I did so, and responses such as yours have been the return."[62]

Barton delivered her appeal for supplies to Archibald Shaver, who was again serving with Barton after taking a year off to recover his failing health. Shaver had 4,500 copies of the document printed at a cost of six dollars and twenty-five cents. For the next two days, Barton and Ferguson addressed copies of the circular to newspaper offices throughout the North.[63] However, it would take at least two weeks for the appeal to bear fruit; in the meantime, soldiers at Fredericksburg were dying for lack of care. Therefore, when Gardiner Tufts suggested that Barton join forces with the Massachusetts state relief agency, she readily agreed. The arrangement benefited both parties. Tufts's agency could use the wagons that Rucker had promised to Barton, while Barton could access Tufts's supplies until she could amass a sufficient quantity of her own.[64]

By May 19, the arrangements necessary for Barton's return to Fredericksburg were falling into place. Wilson had secured from the War Department a pass allowing her to return to the front, the Massachusetts state relief agency had agreed to share its supplies with her when she reached Fredericksburg, and Rucker had promised to provide her with the necessary mules and wagons. Nevertheless, there still remained countless things to do before she left the capital. There were people to write, supplies to purchase, crates to pack. It is little wonder that she was exhausted.[65]

BACK DOWN THE POTOMAC

By May 20, Barton was ready to go. Early in the morning, a wagon rolled up to the Massachusetts state relief agency's warehouse and began loading up crates and barrels of supplies. Barton followed the wagons to the Seventh Street Wharf joined by Shaver, who had agreed to accompany her to Fredericksburg. At the wharf Barton encountered a snag. She found she had no bill of transportation, and officials at the wharf refused to load her goods onto the ship without one. She asked to speak with Captain Allen, the officer in charge. At first, subordinates claimed Allen wasn't in, wrote Barton, "but I produced so many official papers that they concluded he was here & I sent for him. A civilian bystander assured me that he would not come down there. I had best have sent my papers to him, but soon to his consternation the Capt came very fast & my goods were on board."[66]

Barton again took passage on the *Winona*. The ship probably made a stop at Alexandria because it did not reach Belle Plain until 1 P.M. on May 21. On board were several members of the Michigan Soldiers' Relief Association and the wife of Lt. John E. Myers, an officer in the 62nd Pennsylvania. Myers had been shot through the lungs in the Wilderness and was then at a hospital in Fredericksburg. His wife, overwrought with grief and worry, was anxious to reach his side. "She is suffering exceedingly," Barton confided to her diary. "I promised to try to find her a passage to F[rederickburg]."[67]

It took two hours to unload Barton's crates and place them onto wagons for the trip to town. Shaver remained behind at Belle Plain to oversee the operation while Barton started for Fredericksburg in the company of Mrs. Myers, who was frantic to reach her husband. The two ladies persuaded the Michigan relief workers to give them a ride on their wagon, which was piled high with supplies. Although the area's torrential rains had ended four days earlier, the ten-mile journey was still a strain on the horses. To lighten the load, Barton and the others got off and walked when the wagon came to a hill.[68]

At intervals along the way, guards stopped the party to inspect their passes. Secretary Stanton had issued strict orders that no civilians be permitted to travel to Fredericksburg unless they were going there to assist the wounded. The order extended to everyone, even members of Congress.[69] Worried that Shaver did not have a pass, Barton arranged with a captain of the guard to send a messenger back to Captain Pitkin, the assistant quartermaster in charge of transportation at Belle Plain, to secure one for him. She then resumed the toilsome journey, reaching Fredericksburg after dark. The party went directly to the Christian Commission office. Delegates there accompanied Barton to the office of Captain Jones, who rustled up some supper for his guest and arranged for her to stay at the battered home of a family whose husband was in the Confederate army. While Barton sat down to eat, Mrs. Myers hurried off to find her husband. Barton would catch up with her the next day.[70]

Barton spent the night in an upstairs chamber that had been riddled by Union shot and shell during the Battle of Fredericksburg, seventeen months earlier. She did not feel quite safe living in the house of a Southern sympathizer, and as she looked around the room with its scarred walls and sparse furnishings she was distressed to find that there was no way to lock the door: the latch was broken. As she pondered this problem, a small black girl appeared "and insisted upon taking off my boots and rubbing my feet which she did most perfectly." The following morning, as Barton was leaving, she tipped the child fifteen cents. In addition, she paid the owner fifteen cents for the room.[71]

May 22 was a busy day for the Massachusetts native. Unwilling to trust her personal belongings to the care of her Southern hostess, Barton left her satchel with Jones and then sought out Dr. Alfred Hitchcock. Unfortunately, he had left town the previous day. Undaunted, she went in search of J. W. Doe, who appears to have been in charge of the Massachusetts state relief agency workers in town. Doe took her back to his office. By then, it was approaching noon and Barton was tired. She sat down to rest next to a gentleman who seemed to take an unusual interest in her. At length, he asked if she was from Worcester. When Barton acknowledged that she was, the man introduced himself as Dr. Daniel S. Lamb, the twenty-one-year-old brother of Capt. Samuel Lamb, one of her companions back at Hilton Head. Dr. Lamb had come down from Massachusetts ten days earlier to help in the crisis and was now in charge of one of the town's many hospitals. Thrilled at meeting a neighbor so far from home, Barton jumped out of her seat and took him by the hand. "I could not help shedding tears," she recalled. "I scarce knew how to talk. I was so glad to see him, but we *did* talk."[72]

Barton found that she knew other people too. Once her arrival in Fredericksburg became known, she received a message from Edward "Ned" Barton, a cousin who had been traveling with the army as a delegate of the U.S. Sanitary Commission. Struck down by rheumatism early in the campaign, Ned now lay prostrate next to the Baptist church in the parlor of a house owned by a woman named Maria Wolff. Clara briefly visited him there, promising to return later in the day. At that moment, though, she had to return to the Massachusetts state relief agency office. Shaver had arrived from Belle Plain with her supplies, and she needed to meet with him and Doe to unload them. She returned to see Ned later that afternoon. To her surprise, she discovered her traveling companion, Mrs. Myers, in the room adjoining her cousin's. The distraught woman had found her husband alive, but just barely. He was sinking fast and could not speak above a whisper. Within a week he would be dead.[73]

While Clara was visiting with Ned, Fredericksburg's military governor dropped in. Colonel Edmund Schriver, a West Point graduate, had entered the war as lieutenant colonel of the 11th United States Infantry and was later appointed inspector of the Army of the Potomac.[74] He was the most important man in town, and Barton was not above asking him for favors. Producing a letter from Wilson, she asked Schriver if she could apply to the local commissary officer for rations, not only for herself but for the many wounded men she intended to feed. Wilson himself had refused her request for supplies as improper, but Barton felt Schriver might be more compliant. She was wrong. The colonel read the document but concluded that it was a personal letter and carried no official weight. He politely rejected Barton's request.[75]

Leaving Ned to rest, Clara set out to find another cousin, George Barton. George was an ordnance sergeant in the 19th Maine and had been shot through the lungs while fighting in the Wilderness. Captured by the Confederates, he had been held prisoner for fifteen days. A relative had informed Clara that George was in Fredericksburg, but the town was so crowded with wounded men that she didn't know where to find him. By chance, she happened to run into a soldier in the 19th Maine who knew George and was able to lead her to him. Entering the room, she "found a splendid looking fellow,

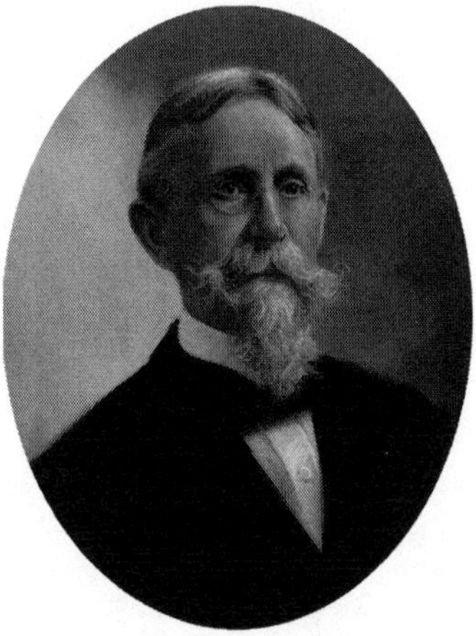

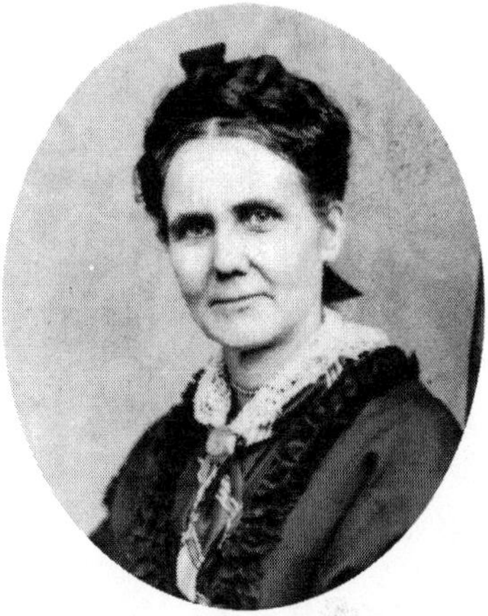

Dr. Daniel S. Lamb, left, as he appeared later in life. (*The National Museum of Health and Medicine, Silver Spring, Maryland*); Isabella Fogg, right. (*Maine State Archives*)

almost a giant," straight and noble. Despite his recent trials, George was up and walking about. The two had a pleasant conversation and parted company only after Clara made him promise to call on her. She returned to her temporary quarters at the Massachusetts state relief agency that afternoon with a light heart.[76]

Her joy increased upon reaching the building, for she found that workers had unpacked her new stove. She put it into operation at once, rustling up a supper of boiled eggs, crackers, toast, and tea for Dr. Lamb and others at the agency, a "little supper" her friends seemed to relish. After the meal, Isabella Fogg stopped in and took tea with the group. Now in her fortieth year, the former seamstress had been serving with the army since the 1862 Peninsula Campaign—longer than even Barton herself. Lamb was Fogg's relative, and he insisted that Barton take Fogg's icebox. Fogg herself went even further, offering to share her quarters with Barton, an offer the newcomer gratefully accepted.[77]

The dishes were still on the table when George Barton entered the room, honoring his earlier pledge to visit Clara at her temporary quarters. Setting aside for a moment the dirty dishes, Clara went with George to see their cousin Ned over by the Baptist church. Later, she returned to the Massachusetts agency and joined the others in clearing the table. As she did so, she heard the whistle of a train across the river at Falmouth Station. The noise "sent a thrill of joy through us all," she wrote, for it meant that the U.S. Military Railroad Construction Corps had finally opened the railroad to Aquia Landing. No more would wounded men have to endure a jolting ten-mile ride over rough corduroy roads to Belle Plain. They could now ride the rails in relative comfort. Later that same day, the first of several light-draft steamships made their way up the Rappahannock River to Fredericksburg. Surgeons could now evacuate wounded soldiers by either train or ship. After two weeks of anguish, the town's medical crisis was finally at an end.[78]

CLARA BARTON BIDS FREDERICKSBURG FAREWELL

With the repair of the railroad to Aquia Landing and the opening of river navigation to Fredericksburg, surgeons could evacuate wounded soldiers to the North efficiently and with little loss of life. They proceeded at once to the task. Surgeon Dalton asked Lamb to escort a party of wounded soldiers to Aquia Landing, and Lamb in turn invited Barton to join him. She agreed, unaware that she would never again return to service with the army.[79]

On May 23, surgeons placed seriously wounded soldiers on ambulances and carried them across the pontoon bridges to Falmouth Station. Attendants then transferred the patients onto railroad cars that carried them to Aquia Landing. Once there, other hands placed the wounded men aboard special ships that carried them up the Potomac River to Washington. Lamb and Barton provided care to the soldiers who made this arduous journey, although to her "it seemed impossible to hold body and soul together till the haven could be gained." In spite of their efforts, several died along the way.[80]

Barton's ship reached Washington on the night of May 24.[81] Back home once more, she finally had time to rest and reflect on the recent campaign. To Mrs. Alling, one of the many people who had responded to her nationwide appeal for supplies, she wrote: "Since the commencement of the war no Campaign has compared with this in magnitude and destruction, and at no time have the arrangements for meeting the necess[i]ties of the field and hospital been so

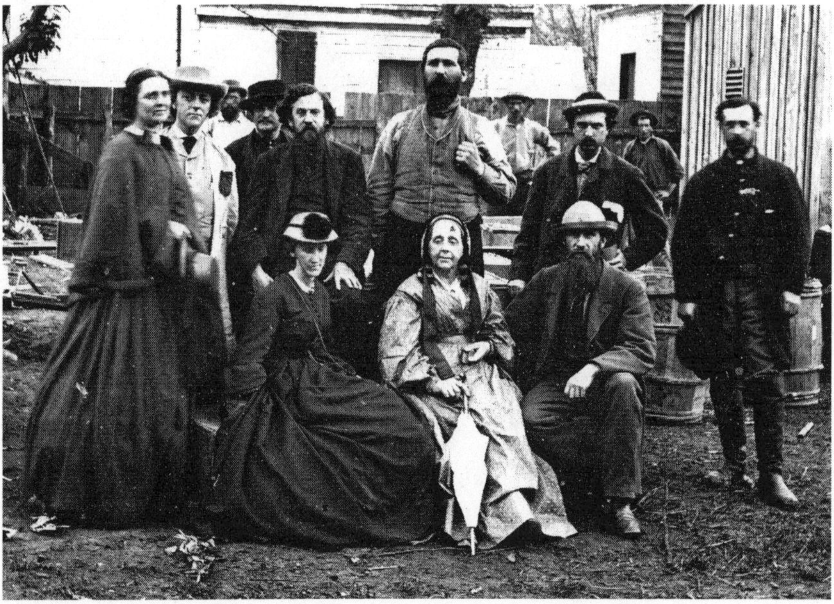

U.S. Sanitary Commission Workers in Fredericksburg, May 1864. (*Library of Congress*)

complete. I cannot express the gratitude I feel, for the noble support vouchsafed, and the successes achieved by the two noble commissions laboring side by side all through the land."[82] Despite such outward praise for the Sanitary and Christian commissions, Barton continued to view them as rivals in the business of battlefield relief. She would cooperate with them and the various state agencies if she had to, but she would never join them. She was too independent for that. Instead, she would continue to play a lone hand, accepting help from such agencies when she needed to, but going it alone when she did not.

6

The Army of the James

"THE TRUE SOLDIER"

Barton was never happier than when she was active and useful. During the three weeks she was in Washington, she kept busy answering correspondence, taking care of personal business, and visiting soldiers in the general hospitals. "I have had but one nights sleep since last thursday," she wrote an acquaintance shortly after returning to the capital. "I had so many personel [*sic*] friends that were mortally wounded, and just reached the city to die. We are waiting at the cotside, and closing their eyes one by one as they pass away. The campaign[,] terrible as it is[,] still looks cheerful and hopeful," she added. "I cannot but think that we shall win at last but *Oh! the cost*—a regiment reduced to a score, and a corporal commanding. Still God demands the sacrifice, and we have only to obey."[1]

Her brother David, fearing that she might fall ill from her incessant labors, advised her to take it easy for a while. Predictably, Clara rejected his advice. "I do not think I shall expose myself to sickness at all," she wrote. "[It] may be [I] shall not go much out from Washington, but I *cannot* keep qu[i]te still, and go off and visit, while this war is going on as it is now. that would not make me *comfortable* at all. I suppose I should feel about as much benefitted as my gold fish would if some kind hearted person should take him out of his vase when he looks so wet and cold and wrap him up in a warm dry flannel. Cant live out of our natural elements can we[?] I'll keep quiet when the war is over," she promised.[2]

By the third week in June, Barton had her affairs in order and was ready to return to the front. By then, the Army of the Potomac had left Fredericksburg, crossed the James River, and laid siege to Petersburg, Virginia. Major General Benjamin F. Butler's Army of the James lay nearby, extending the Union line northward across a broad neck of land known since colonial times as Bermuda Hundred. Butler's army encompassed the Tenth and Eighteenth Corps. The Tenth Corps had come up from South Carolina, and Barton was acquainted with many of its officers, while the Eighteenth Corps consisted of troops that had previously served in North Carolina. With the Sanitary and Christian Commissions strongly represented in the Army of the Potomac, the Army of the James offered a more promising field for Barton's services. Armed with a letter of recommendation from Senator Wilson, she started south in late June to begin work with her fifth military command.[3] It is perhaps a measure of her growing self-confidence that, for the first and only time in the war, she did not feel it necessary to secure the company of a male guardian.

As usual, Barton traveled by ship, taking the *Charlotte Vanderbilt* down the Chesapeake Bay to Fort Monroe, a huge federal installation situated at Old Point Comfort, near Hampton, Virginia. She took advantage of a long layover there to visit Charles Devens, a Massachusetts general who was being treated for inflammatory rheumatism at Chesapeake Hospital. Devens commanded a division in the Eighteenth Corps. There is no evidence that Barton knew the general, but as he was from Massachusetts and a leading general in the Army of the James, she probably felt it was to her advantage to gain his acquaintance.

At 10 A.M. June 22, she reboarded the *Charlotte Vanderbilt* and continued up the James River to City Point, Virginia, the Army of the Potomac's huge supply base located at the mouth of the Appomattox River. When she stepped off the ship at 5 P.M., she recognized the face of her old friend, Capt. Perley Pitkin of the Quartermaster Corps. Pitkin's clerk procured Barton an ambulance and she traveled a short distance to the army's Depot Field Hospital, which was perched on a bluff overlooking the river. There she encountered additional friends, such as Captain James E. Jones of the Quartermaster Corps and Archibald Shaver, her coworker from earlier days. After reporting to Dr. Edward Dalton, she had tea with some of the doctors at the Maine state relief agency before finally settling down at the Massachusetts agency, where, surrounded by old friends, she "felt at home at once." That night, Barton bedded down in a tent with two female relief workers who had just arrived from Ohio. One of the women recalled that their accommodations included grass for a mattress, a log for a pillow, and a "big, war plaid blanket-shawl for a covering." It was an uncomfortable return to army life.[4]

The next morning, June 23, after taking breakfast, Barton returned to the wharf in the company of Col. Charles B. Phillips, of the 130th Ohio. President Lincoln happened to be at City Point that day meeting with Grant, but there is no evidence that Barton knew that he was there, much less that she saw him.[5] Instead, she met with Maj. Gen. Benjamin Butler, the bald, baggy-eyed commander of the Army of the James, who had his headquarters just across the Appomattox River at Bermuda Hundred. Catching a ride across the river on the U.S.S. *Gazelle*, Barton walked a mile from the landing to the general's headquarters and handed him Wilson's letter of introduction. Like Barton, Butler was a Massachusetts native, and he instantly took a liking to her. He not only issued her a pass to move freely throughout the army but also handed her an order directing officers in his command to afford her every facility within their power. She never needed to use either document. "So little inclination do they display to thwart me," she wrote happily, "that I have *never* shown my 'pass and order' to an officer since I have been in the department. I have had but one trouble since I came," she added immodestly, "and that has been to extend my labor without having the point that I leave miss me." Surgeons in both the Army of the Potomac and the Army of the James, she noted, were vying for her services.[6]

THE TENTH CORPS

Perhaps at Butler's suggestion, Barton stopped at the headquarters of Maj. Gen. William T. H. Brooks, who had recently replaced her nemesis, Quincy Gillmore, as commander of the Tenth Corps.[7] The corps had two hospitals: a base hospital located at Point of Rocks and a "flying hospital" situated closer to the front that provided immediate care for soldiers wounded in battle. Like latter-day MASH units, flying hospitals were subject to move at a moment's notice and consequently had to travel light.[8]

At Brooks's headquarters, Barton encountered Surgeon John J. Craven. The Tenth Corps' medical purveyor back in South Carolina, Craven now was serving as its medical director. He and Barton were friends. At his invitation, she established herself at the corps hospital at Point of Rocks. Dr. Horace P. Porter, a surgeon whom Barton described as "a young man of uncommon good nature and ability, enterprising and humane," was in charge of the facility. Although she later claimed that Butler appointed her to be the army's superintendent of nurses, Barton never held that nor any other official position in the army. She was simply a private citizen doing an arduous but important job.[9]

Barton described the corps hospital as "only an overburdened and *well conducted field*" in which "the sufferers were many, and the comforts few."[10] "Some twenty long lines of hospital tents, comprised the hospital," she wrote, "all filled with used up, wounded, worn-out men." Each tent was approximately fifty feet long and had bunks or cots running along each side. For the most part, the Bermuda Hundred line was a static front, and unlike most of her previous assignments Barton's patients consisted not so much of wounded soldiers but of men suffering from ailments incident to camp life such as diarrhea, dysentery, typhoid, measles, and sunstroke. Those with less serious conditions stayed at the hospital for a few days and then returned to their units; other, more serious cases were sent by ship to Fort Monroe and points north. Although it changed daily, the hospital averaged between four hundred and seven hundred patients. Not all of these were men or even adults, for that matter. In September, a fifteen-year-old soldier came to the hospital with a fever. Barton cared for him in her own cabin until the boy's father could come for him. One month later, a German woman who lived in the area appeared seeking treatment for a broken limb. With her came four young children.[11]

On occasion, Barton encountered some of the area's black families. "In all cases they are destitute," she wrote, "having stood the sack of two opposing armies,—what one army left them, the other has taken." A woman who had been a slave on the farm where Barton's hospital stood had no fewer than thirteen children. The owner had fled with the five oldest children at the approach of the Union army. The eight youngest had remained with their mother, who struggled to feed them. Confederate troops had taken the family's bedding and clothing, and the Union troops had taken what little money they had saved. Barton took pity on the family, providing them with food from her kitchen, and used her influence to try and find the mother a job with the army, possibly as a laundress.[12]

Barton's primary responsibility at the hospital was to cook meals for the men—not just the sick and wounded, but also healthy soldiers who had just arrived from Fort Monroe. Sometimes the meals consisted of nothing more than bread and butter; at other times she served fish, rice, pudding, apple pies, donuts—even gingerbread. To men used to subsisting on stale hardtack and salt pork, even the simplest of meals must have seemed like a feast.[13] After each meal Barton had to wash dishes. Then, if time remained, she would visit the wards or return to her tent and write letters.[14]

The days were long; the work, hard. Barton not only cooked for the soldiers, she gave them things necessary for their comfort, oversaw their bathing and care, kept vigil at the bedsides of those who were dying, and attended the funerals of those she could not save.[15] Some idea of a typical day can be gleaned from a letter she wrote to a friend in Washington. "Please tell the noble ladies of New York," she wrote, "that less than an hour ago I blistered my hands spreading their hard, sweet, yellow butter on to sliced bread for five hundred and fifty men's suppers. I remember when it was quite an item to make the yearly barrel of 'apple sauce' for family use. I have had a barrel made to-day, and given out every spoonful of it with my own hands. I have cooked ten dozen eggs, made cracker toast, corn starch, blanc mange, milk punch, arrow-root, washed faces and hands, put ice on hot heads, mustard on cold feet, written six 'soldiers' letters home,' stood beside three death-beds . . . and now, at this hour, midnight, I am too sleepy and stupid to write even you a tolerably readable scrap. It has been a long day, and the mercury is at something over a hundred, and no breeze."[16]

As Barton's letter attests, the summer of 1864 was unusually hot and dry, even by Virginia standards, leading to many cases of sunstroke. Week after week passed without rain, and dust choked the land. Writing in early July, she noted, "This has been one of the hottest days I ever knew. The whole country is parched like a heap of ashes; there is not even dew; the fields are crisp, and the corn leaves curling, as if under flame." As usual, it was the patients who suffered most. "It is terribly oppressive for the sick, painful for the wounded," she wrote, "and still I dare not pray for rain. This hot breath of devastation sweeps over the fruitful fields, and destroys the substance of our enemies. It is worth more than battles, and we must not only endure it, but thank God and take courage." Writing one day later, she observed: "The same hot glare, not a ripple on the river, not a leaf stirs." As the summer advanced, things would only get worse.[17]

Barton did not run the hospital alone. In addition to Dr. Porter, she labored beside Assistant Surgeon Edward F. Dodge of the 19th Wisconsin; a hospital steward named Mann, who owned an intelligent little terrier; and a sixty-eight-year-old ward master of Spanish descent named Thomas Don Carlos, a man she considered "clear, true, warm hearted & dignified."[18] In late July, the army's medical director augmented the hospital staff by assigning to it four nurses headed by thirty-three-year-old Adelaide W. Smith. The group had been trained by Sarah P. Edson. Like Barton, Edson had served as an independent nurse early in the war. In 1862, she conceived the idea of opening a home where she could train volunteer nurses before they went to the front and where, if necessary, they could withdraw from their labors and rest. With the financial backing of the Masons, she created the Army Nurses' Association in 1863, establishing her training center at Clinton Hall, New York. In 1864, her nurses began taking the field.[19]

Barton clashed with Edson's nurses from the start. A Confederate raid on Washington in July had prompted the District of Columbia resident to rush home to check on her belongings. Edson's nurses arrived while she was gone. Their leader, Adelaide Smith, had come to Bermuda Hundred in the belief that she would be replacing Barton, only to discover upon her arrival that Barton would be returning. Surgeon Porter nevertheless invited Smith and her nurses to stay until Barton came back. When Barton appeared at Point of Rocks on July 31, she found Smith and her followers working in the hospital. Although Barton greeted the newcomers cordially, Smith could see at once that she was not pleased. To add to Barton's displeasure, she discovered that her friend, the "Old Spaniard," Don Carlos, had left the department while she was away. Without him, the hospital would no longer seem the same.[20]

As so often happened when things did not go her way, Barton sulked. On August 6, she confided to her diary: "I cannot feel rightly and do little or nothing. . . . Some complaints begin to come in from Mrs[.] Edson's nurses; I am very sorry they ever came. I hear, but dare not say much." The next day was no better. "Still do not feel free," she wrote. "Cramped & unhappy. Miss Old Uncle Don." Tensions increased when Smith's nurses started bickering among themselves and complaining about everyone else. "Still unhappy," wrote Barton, "Nurses still differing. Miss S. still domineering[.] Still regret Mrs. Edson's visit, and do not believe in Missions."[21]

If Barton wasn't impressed with the new nurses, neither were they impressed with her. Steeped in self-pity, Barton did little work and when asked to help, did so grudgingly. Smith recalled running to the New Englander's tent one day to get bandages for surgeons who were engaged in an operation. Rather than fetch the items quickly, Barton purposely dragged her feet. "She asked about my health," Smith recalled, "urged me to take a seat, and very slowly rummaged about for the necessary supplies. The only time I saw her actively engaged," the new nurse insisted, "was on a day when there had been a skirmish at the front, and she started for the field with the ambulance and an orderly, and a small box of bandages, condensed milk, etc." One day, Barton overheard Smith complaining to Porter about her lack of cooperation. That was the last straw. Striding into the medical director's tent, she told the surgeon that she could no longer work beside Smith and her nurses and wished to leave. Porter wouldn't hear of it, however, and instead transferred the newcomers across the Appomattox River to the Depot Field Hospital. As they left, Smith bid Barton a frosty good-bye.[22]

Barton's rift with Smith was predictable, for she did not work well with other women. At any point during the war, she could have aligned herself with the U.S. Sanitary Commission or other relief organizations that accepted female workers, but she always chose to remain autonomous. In part, this was due to her independent spirit. She liked being in charge and found it hard to take orders from others. But there was another reason: jealousy. Barton viewed the officers and soldiers with whom she worked as her special charges—her family—and she resented sharing their affection and gratitude with others, particularly if the others were women younger and more attractive than herself. She made her feelings on the subject clear in a letter written one year earlier to her cousin Elvira Stone when Stone suggested that she take on a female assistant. Although Barton tried to make a virtue of her objections, it's clear that she simply didn't want any competition.[23]

> You speak of an assistant for me,—while I appreciate the kindly offer, it will be necessary for me to say, as I have at least a hundred times before under similar circumstances that the nature of my position admits of no lady assistant; my own *conscience* would not admit of it.—How could I answer to myself, if I permitted a young lady to leave home and loving friends, & come to me, knowing nothing of the horrors and dangers of field life and place herself unsuspectingly in the immediate jaws of death, or mutilation worse than death.—how shall I answer to those *friends*?! My position is one of my own choosing, full of hardship, and fraught with danger, one that *I* could not have chosen, if I had had father or mother, or husband, or child, or even brothers or sisters whose interests centered at all in *me*, in whose home or family circles my absense [*sic*] would leave a vacuum, at whose fireside my loss would leave a painful void.—I am singularly free. —there are few to mourn for me, and I take my life in my hand and go where men fall and die, to see if perchance I can render some little comfort as the wife or mother would if she could be there.—I know nothing of hospitals,—nothing of security, nothing of permanency, nothing of remuneration, but *give* all I have of

> time[,] strength and means, and give it directly to those who need, and reserve nothing to even help *sustain* an assistant if I had one. —my own living on Morris Island all the time I was there, and will be again when I return[,] was what the soldiers call "salt junk," old beef of such hardness and salt[i]ness as you never dreamed of, lean bacon, and hard crackers, both buggy and wormy. there was not a potato or other cooking vegetable on that island for weeks. . . . The men worked *sixteen hours* in twenty four in the midst of fire and death to hold the enemy *back.*— twenty four hours, that he could not raise his head erect once, could only be relieved under cover of darkness, and all this with a little peice [*sic*] of salt meat and four wormy crackers in his *pocket*, and a canteen of warm water, and when wounded and bro[ugh]t in if I had a mouthful of soft or palatable food to give him, it looked brighter to me than gold, and no mouthful of it passed my lips, or ever could until there was enough for *all*; now this is a hard look for a young lady assistant is it not?[24]

On the rare occasions when Barton did accept female assistants, she took great pains to make sure that they did not outshine her, selecting only those with limited physical appeal. Colonel Alvin Voris thought it a wise policy. After all, he mused, Barton didn't want her assistants to "fall from grace, or bring the sisters of the Army into any danger of departure from the most virtuous walk with God and man" by having illicit relationships with the soldiers. The best way to accomplish that, he reasoned, was to hire women with plain faces. Such a policy benefitted Barton too, for she shined by comparison.[25] In fact, the thirty-seven-year-old Voris thought Barton "the only lady I have seen worth seeing since I came to the Hundred." He went on to describe her as having a large head, strong features, black hair sprinkled with gray, well-developed muscles, and a dark complexion. In personality, he found her "afraid to contradict, kind in manner, easy of address and unaffected & frank in action." "Lord! what a woman," he exclaimed. Barton would have blushed with delight to know that Voris believed her to be just thirty-two years of age (in fact, she was then nearly forty-three), but at the same time she might have furrowed her brow had she read that, while the colonel thought her a "good girl," he also considered her "a little odd."[26]

THE CRATER

Barton had a knack of reaching the front just as a battle was taking place. She had arrived at Antietam on the night of September 16, 1862, fewer than twelve hours before the fighting there started; she had docked off Hilton Head on April 7, 1863, just as Union ironclads began their attack on Fort Sumter; and her ship had dropped anchor at Belle Plain on May 12, amid the struggle for Spotsylvania's "Bloody Angle." Barton was no fatalist, but she did find the coincidence strange. "I had never missed of finding the trouble I went to find," she later wrote, "and was never late."[27] Her return to Point of Rocks after visiting Washington likewise coincided with a battle. The day she stepped off the ship, July 30, Union soldiers detonated a mine under a section of the Confederate line east of Petersburg, igniting what became known as the Battle of the Crater. In the fighting that ensued, the Ninth Corps sustained heavy casualties. Barton's friend J. W. Doe arrived at Point of Rocks two days later with news of the battle, including the names of several of Barton's friends who had been casualties in the fight. Sergeant Horace Gardner was dead, Capt. William H. Clark wounded, and Col. Jacob P. Gould had lost a limb. The list went on, Barton wrote, but "I was too sad to desire to hear more. . . . All that I had feared so long had transpired and I was not near by" to help. "Could have done nothing if I had been," she reflected. That night she mounted a horse and rode to City Point and visited the Ninth Corps hospital early the next day in the company of her friend Doe. After chatting with Gould, Clark, and others, she returned to Point of Rocks with Surgeon Whitman V. White of the 57th Massachusetts.[28]

Her diary says as much. In later years, however, Barton told a much different story. At a reunion of the 21st Massachusetts, she insisted that the regiment had sent a troop of horsemen to tell her the news. Immediately mounting a horse, she rode twenty miles through the night amid a fearful thunderstorm—not to City Point, but to the Crater itself. "At the mine, we found everything in confusion," she told her listeners. "Toward the last of the second day we were there we received news that the enemy had buried the Union dead. We had only to go back as it was." In reality, confusion at the Crater had subsided long before Barton left Point of Rocks. And she could not have inspected the Crater, except from a distance, for the simple reason that it continued to be held by the Confederates. Barton might have known all this had she actually visited the Crater, but she did not.[29]

She *was* at the scene of another explosion, however. On August 8, she accompanied two surgeons from her hospital to visit the U.S.S. *Matilda*, a ship anchored at City Point. They went there to pick up supplies for the hospital, returning with hundreds of sheets, shirts, pillowcases, and other linen items.[30] The following day, a Confederate saboteur slipped a homemade bomb onto a gunpowder barge moored at the ordnance wharf. The resulting explosion killed at least forty-three people and caused $2 million in damage.[31] Barton later told a friend, with only slight exaggeration, that she left the dock "*just in time* to avoid that terrible catastrophy [*sic*]. I was not blown to atoms but might have been and no one the wiser."[32]

No sooner had Barton returned from her trip to City Point than the Tenth Corps was ordered across the James River to attack Richmond. Even if the gambit did not succeed, it would draw Confederate troops away from Petersburg, allowing the Army of the Potomac to capture the Weldon Railroad, south of the city. In preparation for the movement, five hundred sick and wounded soldiers transferred from their regimental hospitals to the Tenth Corps hospital, boosting the number of patients there to twelve hundred. "Only think of such an addition to a family between supper and breakfast and no preparation," Barton wrote. If the huge influx of new patients wasn't bad enough, both her cook and assistant cook happened to be sick at the time, forcing Barton to step into the breach and manage the cooking herself. At one breakfast alone she served seven hundred loaves of bread, 170 gallons of coffee, "two large wash boilers full of tea," a barrel of applesauce and another of boiled pork, half a barrel of blanc-mange (a dessert made of milk, cream, and sugar thickened with corn starch), five hundred slices of buttered toast, a hundred slices of broiled steak, plus enough chicken gruel and boiled eggs to feed 150 patients who could not eat more solid food. On some days she made apple pies for the soldiers under her care; on others, gingerbread or donuts—all on a staggering scale. "Oh what a volume it would make if I could only write you what I have seen, known, heard, and done since I first came to this dept.," she wrote her friend. "The most surprising of all of which is . . . that I should have *turned cook*. Who would have 'thunk it'?"[33]

The August 1864 attack against Richmond failed, but Grant was undeterred. Six weeks later, he again sent Butler's army across the James River to menace Richmond, this time in an effort to prevent Lee from dispatching reinforcements to the Shenandoah Valley. On September 29, Federal troops captured Fort Harrison, a key stronghold just seven miles outside the city. Lee counterattacked but was unable to retake the ground. To support the offensive, Butler ordered Porter to move the base hospital from Point of Rocks across the Bermuda Hundred Peninsula to Jones's Landing on the James River.[34] Barton took an ironclad monitor upriver to the landing and distributed food to soldiers at the flying hospital, which stood nearby. Over the next few days she prepared food at one or both of the hospitals. When she wasn't cooking, she helped lay out the grounds of the new base hospital and supervised the erection of its tents. Shelter for women was scarce, and on October 12, when an officer's wife decided to share Barton's tent without her permission, Barton's patience snapped. She resigned her position at the base hospital, commenting that the intruder was "very welcome to my room, but not my companionship."[35] Once again, she showed her inability to work with, or even tolerate, other women.

Barton left the base hospital but not the army. Instead, she took up residence at the Tenth Corps flying hospital, then under the supervision of Surgeon Martin S. Kittinger of the 100th New York, an acquaintance from her South Carolina days. In no time at all she found herself up to her ears in "confusion, excitement, and hard labor," and she loved every minute of it. "My vineyard has been large, and I have labored hard," she enthusiastically told some of those who contributed to her efforts. "Others may have wrought to much greater purpose but few I trust more earnestly or happily." As a result of her duties, she was unable to respond to letters as promptly as she would have liked. "I have been too busy to speak," Barton explained to her cousin Elvira Stone, "even to my friends since last April, and I am just as busy still, not a moment that I find myself at leisure. And still I leave *so much* undone . . . but one thing

I am certain of, I have labored up to the full measure of my strength. All summer my field has been broad. . . . I cannot tell you how many times I have moved with my whole family of a thousand or fifteen hundred, and with a half hours notice in the night perhaps, sometimes under the guns & no time to waste."[36] In an effort to impress her cousin, Barton grossly exaggerated the number of times she had had to pack up and move. At the time she wrote this letter, she had been with the flying hospital little more than a week.[37]

STEPHEN BARTON

Soon after her arrival at the flying hospital Barton received disturbing news that Union troops had captured her brother Stephen and placed him under guard at Norfolk, Virginia. Eight years earlier Stephen had left Massachusetts to seek his fortune on the North Carolina coast. He purchased a sawmill on the Chowan River and established a community around it called Bartonville. To the sawmill he later added a post office, gristmill, lumberyard, and several warehouses.[38] When the war began, Stephen remained in North Carolina to protect his property despite pleas from Clara that he return to Massachusetts.[39] For three years, he did his best to remain neutral, trading cotton to Union gunboats that prowled the Chowan in return for much-needed foodstuffs, which he sold at a profit in Petersburg.[40] However, his luck ran out on September 25, 1864. While on his way to South Mills, he ran into a Union patrol that questioned him about his dealings with a man named Harney, who was then standing trial in Norfolk for smuggling. A detective traveling with the patrol ordered Stephen to go to Norfolk and be a witness at the trial and then proceeded to take from Stephen every cent that he had on him—a total of more than $2,300. He promised to return the money when Stephen caught up with him again at Norfolk.[41]

Stephen met the patrol at the appointed location, but instead of returning his money the detective confiscated Stephen's horse and wagon and had him confined in a filthy guardhouse where he languished for eighteen days on a bare floor without proper food, blankets, or medicine. "It *may* be that love of country alone incited these young officers to such a course, or rendered such stringent measures necessary in their judgment," Clara wrote skeptically, "but these are *facts*—viz. that he was to all appearance an old man, weak and sick, failing every day, and in case he *should die* in their hands, it was doubtful if any *successful claimant* would appear for the moneys taken from him—or for the team, and lading worth in all some 3,500, or 4000" dollars.[42]

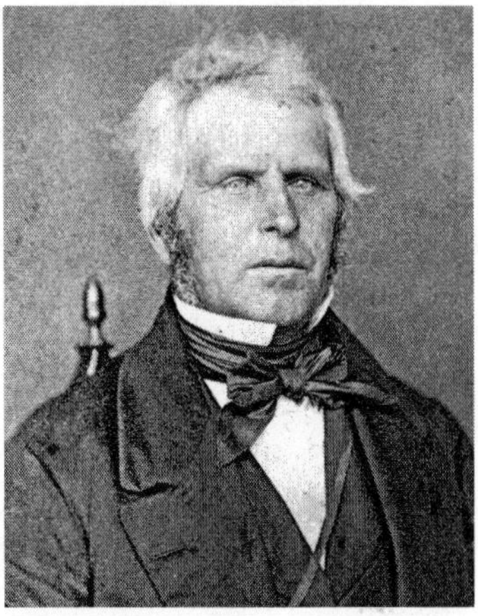

Stephen Barton, Jr., Clara's eldest brother (*Library of Congress*)

Fortunately, Stephen managed to get Clara word of his predicament, and she used her influence with Butler to have him brought to Bermuda Hundred, where the general could personally examine his case. When Stephen arrived on October 25, he was in bad shape. Although just fifty-eight years old, he had chronic diarrhea and was suffering from chills and fever. Clara was shocked at his appearance. "Six years before I had seen Stephen, strong, muscular, erect, two hundred pounds," she wrote. "He walked into my presence now, pale, tottering, a hundred and thirty, his thin white locks resting upon his shoulders, bent and walking feebly with a cane."[43]

To protect her brother from the elements, Clara took over a "log shanty" formerly belonging to a slave and transformed it into a "cozy little house." "When I took it ten days ago," she told Elvira Stone, "it had neither floor, shelf or window; now it has all these & a chamber with real stairs, both floors carpeted with army blankets, the walls papered with newspaper, a good lounge, a wide bed, two tables, closet, stuff[ed] rocking chair[,] wood box, oil cloth hearth rug, and an arbor all the way around it. My chimney is on the outside, being larger than the house, but Oh! what a fire is blazing in it." Clara put Stephen to bed in a room upstairs and arranged for him to have a private nurse. She took the downstairs room for herself. "With all our care we *may not* be able to raise him from his present debilitated condition," she informed her cousin, "but be that as it may, I shall be content to know that he does not lay his bones on alien soil[,] to know at last that he was true to the land that gave him birth and nurtured him."[44]

Stephen was tried by a military court in November and acquitted of the charges against him, but physically he continued to decline. If it was not enough to care for the hundreds of soldiers in her hospital, Clara now had to nurse her brother too. The double duty took its toll on her spirits. She described to a relative her weeks of "labor, anxiety, [and] weariness," and of her "alternating hope and fear" as she stood "over Stephen's sick bed day & night . . . soothing him under all perplexities" and "cheering him under his despondency. . . . All this added to the cares of a hospital in the front of a fighting army, liable to break up at any moment. . . . I have not seen the face of a woman, white or black for months," she wrote with some exaggeration, "walking on blistered feet every day and falling asleep any hour, per sheer necessity some time in the night—all these things have made me a little earnest and sometimes I have wickedly or foolishly felt that it was time I was relieved by other friends. But I know the true soldier stands patiently at his post, no matter what betide, and I will try to, and hold out faithfully to the end." As cold weather set in, Clara sent Stephen back to Washington to be cared for by their sister, Sally Vassell. Before long she would follow.[45]

THE TWENTY-FOURTH CORPS

Late in the year, the Army of the James underwent reorganization. The War Department abolished the Tenth and Eighteenth Corps and replaced them with the all-white Twenty-fourth Corps and the all-black Twenty-fifth Corps. Barton worked at the flying hospital of the Twenty-fourth Corps, but occasionally she had an opportunity to see and meet soldiers of the Twenty-fifth. In a letter written for publication a few months earlier, she had gone out of her way to praise the black soldiers. "They are ever the objects of my deep commiseration and care," she had written in July, "so patient and cheerful, so uniformly polite and soldierly. They are brave men and make no complaints, and yet I cannot pass one without the keenest desire to give him something; and it is enough they need, poor fellows. One feature especially pleases me, the excellent nurses they make, and the kind care they take of each other, in camp and hospital. But I am well satisfied that they are not a class of men that an enemy would desire to meet on a charge. They have wants as soldiers now, as well as 'Freedmen,' and I sincerely hope this fact may not be overlooked by their northern friends."[46]

As this letter indicates, Barton's views on slavery had evolved significantly during the war. Prior to that time, she had viewed slaves as useless to the country, fit only "for missionary labors and candidates for eternity," but contact with Frances D. Gage had changed her mind. Barton had met Gage in South Carolina, where she found Gage laboring without pay among the former slaves on Parris Island. Although the Ohio native was thirteen years older than Barton, the two women had much in common. Both had been raised in the Universalist Church, both had been tomboys in their youth, both were activists with strong feminist views, and both enjoyed poetry. They quickly became close friends. In her letters and conversations with Barton, Gage impressed upon her friend the evils of slavery and the dignity of blacks as human beings. Gage's views coincided with Barton's own observations. While serving in the South, Barton had seen and spoken with many former slaves, and she must have admired their fortitude in the face of adversity. She was particularly impressed with the black men serving as soldiers in the army, whom she found both courageous and uncomplaining. "Whiter blood than their's has often failed to exhibit traits as high and noble," she opined in a letter written for publication.[47]

While Barton admired the black troops, her first responsibility was to the men of her own corps. In a letter to her relative Annie Childs, Barton appealed for additional supplies of food and clothing. Winter was coming on, she warned, and many of the relief workers soon would be leaving to enjoy the comforts of home. "Nevertheless the troops will need the same care, good warm shirts, socks, drawers, and mittens, and the sick will need the same good, well-cooked diet that they did in summer; and yet it would try me dreadfully to be among them in the cold and nothing comfortable to give them. And this corps especially never passed a winter north of South Carolina and they *will nearly freeze*, I fear. I have scraped together and given already the last warm article I have just for the few frosty nights we have had. I haven't a pair of socks or shirts or drawers for a soldier in my possession. I shall look with great anxiety now for anything to reach me, for I shall require it both on account of the increased severity of the weather and my proposed extended field of labor." The extended field of labor mentioned by Barton consisted of supplying *all* the patients in her corps, both those at the base hospital and at the flying hospital. She felt uniquely qualified to do this, having worked at both facilities. "I could keep the needy portion of a whole corps comfortably supplied; and being connected with the hospital and convalescent camp, conversant with the men, surgeons, and nurses, I could meet their wants more timely and surely than any stranger or outside organization of men could do," she explained.[48]

Barton's plans to supply the men of both hospitals never came to fruition. Instead, as the calendar page turned to 1865 she continued to find herself in charge of cooking operations at the Twenty-fourth Corps flying hospital, which occupied the grounds of a plantation one mile from Dutch Gap. The surgeons and their assistants occupied the plantation house itself, the outbuildings functioned as storehouses for the hospital, and Barton shared the slave cabins west of the mansion with members of the Sanitary and Christian Commissions. A fifteen-foot-tall fence made of pine trees set close together surrounded Barton's cabin, concealing it from view. According to Stephen, Clara's friends fitted up the cabin "in superb style," building her a brick chimney, papering her interior walls, and even carpeting her floors. Her kitchen stood twenty feet west of the cabin. Consisting of two tents, it fairly bulged with boxes and barrels of food delivered each day from the base hospital. Four stockades, each fifty feet in length and covered with canvas, constituted the wards.[49]

With the approach of winter, Clara's life became more settled. Stephen described her daily routine: "She arises in the morning about 6 1/2 o'clock," he told relatives,

> goes in to the cooking tent and directs the cooks in preparing the light diet for the more feeble of the sick and wounded soldiers whose many wants take her attention until after 8 o'clock. She takes all her meals at the surgeon's table. Breakfast at 8 1/2 and dinner at 3 o'clock and no supper. Her time between the two meals she generally spends directing the business in her cooking tent, gets through with serving out the delicacies which those sick and

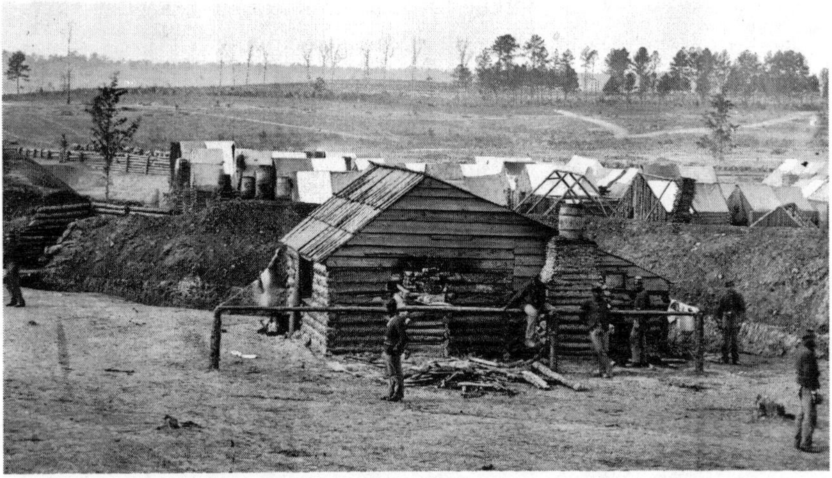

Fort Burnham. Both Union and Confederate pickets are visible in this remarkable image, just as Barton described them. (*Library of Congress*)

> feeble men require about 6 p.m. She then comes in to her house and attends to her correspondence which often takes her until late bed time. She rides on horseback one afternoon in each week about 6 miles to the base hospital situated on the river where [are stored] all the boxes and Barrels of food that are constantly reaching her from the charitable people of our yet great nation. This is her regular routine of business, besides she attends numerous calls each day from her friends and acquaintances.[50]

Among those who paid calls on Barton was Col. Alvin Voris, whom Barton had met in South Carolina. As she did with many of the officers, Barton shared with Voris small items of food from her larder—things such as apples, eggs, butter, and pies. He responded to these "little acts of kindness" by detailing some of his men to fix up her cabin for the winter. Soon the two were good friends. On December 4, they took a ride together up to the front, Barton riding a "wicked horse" called Rob. "I said all my funny, winning sayings in my best style," Voris told his wife, and "she like a polite lady said yes to everything." He and Barton rode to Fort Burnham, took a look at the rebel pickets visible in the distance, and then rode back along the lines to Barton's cabin. "Miss Barton is a real good woman,"

Voris concluded, "full of kindness of heart." His friendship with her would outlast the war.[51]

With military affairs in front of Richmond and Petersburg at a temporary impasse, Grant turned his attention to Fort Fisher, located near the mouth of the Cape Fear River. The fort protected Wilmington, North Carolina, the Confederacy's last open port. If he could reduce Fort Fisher and capture Wilmington, he would effectively cut the South off from the outside world. Grant assigned Butler the task of taking the fort, but Barton's friend botched the job. Undeterred, Grant ordered another attack, this time led by Maj. Gen. Alfred H. Terry, now in charge of the Twenty-fourth Corps. Barton wanted to accompany Terry's expedition, but she was not asked to come.[52]

By the time Terry's forces captured Fort Fisher, Barton was no longer in Virginia. Butler's failure to capture the fort led Grant to relieve him of command on January 8, 1865. At the same time, Barton's "old true and tried friend," Dr. Kittinger, announced that he would soon be resigning his position as head of the flying hospital and going home.[53] Those two developments, coupled with her concern over Stephen's health, prompted Barton to return to Washington for the winter. Before leaving, however, she decided to make one last tour of the front lines and say good-bye to friends. Between January 9 and 12 she visited Fort Harrison, which Union troops had captured back in September and rechristened Fort Burnham. Hostile cannons in a nearby Confederate fort frowned down upon the work, while a just a few hundred yards away, in clear sight, stood a line of rebel pickets. Despite these threats, Barton found soldiers of the Seventh United States Colored Troops busily at work on a log building that they intended to use as both chapel and schoolhouse. "Talk no more of fiction," she scribbled in her diary, "truth is far more striking and strange. Work on poor fellows, God is with you."[54]

Upon returning from the three-day excursion, Barton distributed her remaining supplies among the patients and made arrangements to leave. At 4 p.m., January 12, 1865, she rode with Kittinger and a man named Brown to Varina Landing, where they caught a ride across the James River to Bermuda Hundred. Barton and her small party spent the night aboard the U.S.S. *James T. Brady*, a mail boat that was leaving for Washington the next day. The ship made a stop at Fort Monroe and then proceeded on to the capital, which it reached around noon, January 14.[55] Barton planned to be away for just a few months, and when Kittinger's successor begged her to return to the flying hospital she promised that she would. But she would not keep that vow. Before she returned, Grant would mount a spring offensive that would break Lee's lines and compel him to surrender. Barton's days in the army were over.[56]

7

Later Years

"THE PATHS OF CHARITY"

Once in the nation's capital, Clara Barton discharged some overdue bills, paid social calls on friends, and caught up on back correspondence, not only with friends and relatives but also with people and organizations that supported her work. She had frequent meetings with Senator Wilson and others regarding the introduction of a bill increasing the rank of army surgeons. Between these and other activities she found time to attend a White House levee hosted by Mary Todd Lincoln.[1] However, it was Stephen's health that remained uppermost in her mind. Her fifty-eight-year-old brother was still "quite feeble" in her estimation; in fact, if anything, his condition had grown worse since leaving Virginia, possibly the result of his having applied what Clara considered to be "injudicious remedies."[2] Although Stephen had been acquitted of charges of illegal trading in November, the government still had not released his property, and on February 1, 1865, Clara sailed to Norfolk on her brother's behalf in hopes of resolving the matter. She had several interviews with the city's provost marshal about Stephen's case and met socially with Gens. Israel Vodges and Newton M. Curtis, both of whom had commanded brigades in the Tenth Corps.[3]

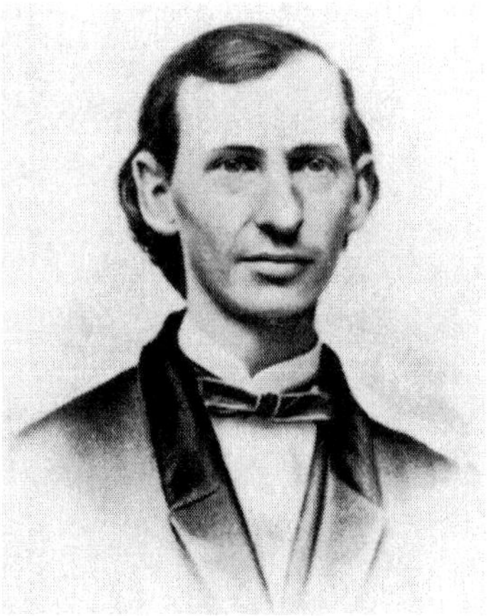

Irving Vassall.
(*Library of Congress*)

Barton returned to Washington via Annapolis, Maryland, on February 10. While awaiting a train at Annapolis Junction she happened to run into Dorothea Dix, the Superintendent of Army Nurses, whose minions had given Barton so much annoyance in South Carolina. Then sixty-two years of age, Dix had gained fame prior to the war for her work in creating humane asylums for the mentally ill. At one time Barton probably admired her; now she viewed her as a rival. Nevertheless, on the surface the two behaved cordially, exchanging cards and promising to call on one another in the future. They never did.[4]

Back in Washington, Barton hurried to the home of her sister, Sally Vassall, where she found her brother Stephen "weaker than I left him."[5] Just as alarming, Sally's son Irving was ill too. A clerk under Gardiner Tufts at the Massachusetts state relief agency in Washington, Irving had been battling tuberculosis for some time, and it was finally getting the better of him. Barton had planned to fulfill her pledge and return to her flying hospital on the James—in fact, she had even gone so far as to have her field dress taken in and trimmed with plaid—but with both Stephen and Irving in precarious health, she put aside those plans and remained in Washington. Family came first.[6]

Stephen soon succumbed to his illness. On March 10, Clara wrote in her diary, "God took our poor dear brother from his cares and troubles." She was with him when he died. "Did our mother welcome him[?]" she wondered. "Oh! the thin, strong veil, when shall it fall that we may see?"[7] Clara sent Stephen's body back to Massachusetts for burial and then traveled north herself to attend the funeral.[8] One month later, on April 9, Irving too died. He had been Clara's favorite nephew, and his demise, coming on the heels of Stephen's death, dealt her a staggering blow, one that not even the surrender of Lee's army, which occurred that same day, could assuage. Months later, she privately reflected on her dual loss. "Within these 12 months I have parted with the two who perhaps in the old time has twined the most deeply about my heart, who had traits of character more in common with myself than any others, where love for me was a mine of wealth, and around whose dear morning the tenderest fibres of my heart still cling[,] and crushed & torn, and buried still ache and bleed."[9]

Characteristically, Barton dealt with her grief by pitching into her work. With the war winding down she no longer was needed at the front, so instead she embarked on a new project: helping Northern families track down their missing relatives in the army. Each year thousands of Union soldiers had simply vanished from the rolls. Some had died on the field of battle, others had perished in hospitals or in Southern prisons, a few deserted. Because the government did not issue death notices, thousands of Northern families remained in doubt as to the fate of loved ones who did not return home. In their anguish some people had written to Barton, hoping to gain information about missing husbands and sons. In the past she had been too busy to reply to their inquiries, but now she saw an opportunity to help. At Annapolis, Union authorities had established a camp for paroled Union prisoners awaiting exchange.[10] These men had just come from Southern prisons and undoubtedly had valuable information about comrades, living and dead, whom they had left behind. Someone simply had to gather, organize, and distribute that information, and Barton felt that she was the one to do it. Henry Wilson brought the project to the attention of President Lincoln, who in turn referred the matter to Maj. Gen. Ethan A. Hitchcock, the Commissary General of Prisoners.[11] Hitchcock supported the idea, and within a matter of days Barton issued the following announcement in a local newspaper:

> PAROLED AND EXCHANGED PRISONERS.
> In view of the great anxiety felt throughout the country for the welfare of our prisoners now being exchanged, and arriving at Annapolis, Maryland, Miss Clara Barton, by permission of Gen. Hitchcock, Commissioner of Exchange, with the sanction of the President, has kindly undertaken to furnish information by

> correspondence in regard to the condition of returned soldiers, especially those in the hospitals at Annapolis and also as far [as] possible to learn the facts in reference to those that have died in prison, or elsewhere. All letters addressed to Miss Clara Barton, Annapolis, Maryland, will meet with prompt attention. Editors throughout the country are requested to copy this notice.[12]

As news of Barton's endeavor spread throughout the country, inquiries began to arrive by the thousands. Barton transferred the Missing Soldiers Office, as she called her enterprise, to her Washington, D.C., residence. From there, she issued lists containing the names of missing soldiers to newspapers and post offices throughout the country, asking anyone with information about those men to write to her. She then passed the information she received on to the soldiers' families. It was a worthy project, but insufficient funding and the lack of official recognition by the War Department ultimately compelled Barton to close her doors in 1867. Nevertheless, during the short time the office was open, she claimed to have answered 63,182 letters and identified more than 22,000 men.[13]

THE ANDERSONVILLE EXPEDITION

More than half of Barton's identifications came from a single source: Private Dorence Atwater. Atwater had enlisted in the 2nd New York Cavalry at the age of sixteen only to be captured after the Battle of Gettysburg. While detailed by his captors as a clerk in the surgeon's office at the notorious Confederate prison camp in Andersonville, Georgia, he had secretly copied a register listing the names and burial locations of some 13,000 Union soldiers who had died there. When finally exchanged in March 1865, he successfully smuggled the document back north and shared its contents with the government in return for $300 and a position as clerk in the War Department.[14]

Atwater meanwhile had learned of Barton's efforts to locate missing soldiers and offered her his assistance.[15] When he told her about the Andersonville register, Barton appealed to Bvt. Maj. Gen. William Hoffman, the Commissary General of Prisoners, to send a party to Andersonville at once to identify and mark the graves. Secretary of War Stanton approved the idea and directed Assistant Quartermaster James M. Moore to lead the expedition.[16] A

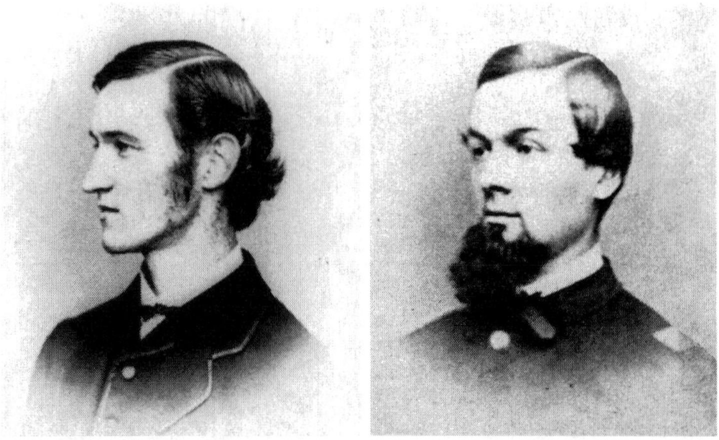

Dorence Atwater, left, and Captain James Moore, right. (*Library of Congress*)

Pennsylvanian by birth, Moore had enlisted in the army as a private and had risen steadily through the ranks to become a brevet major by war's end. Along the way, he had switched to the quartermaster corps, where he became a specialist in the identification and burial of the dead.[17] Because Atwater was familiar with Andersonville and its cemetery, Stanton ordered him to accompany Moore's party. He invited Barton to go along too, perhaps because she had proposed the idea.[18] Forty workmen completed the party. With them they took fencing materials to enclose the cemetery grounds, seven thousand unlettered pine headboards, and the tools necessary to complete the job.[19]

The party departed Washington on July 8, 1865, aboard the steamship *Virginia* and headed for Savannah, Georgia.[20] The trip got off to a rocky start when the ambulance sent by Moore to get Barton arrived five hours late. For some reason, Moore blamed Barton for the delay. As soon as she arrived, he stormed on deck and exclaimed angrily for all to hear, "G-d damn it to hell! Some people don't deserve to go anywhere, and what in Hell does she want to go for?" The verbal assault left Barton stunned and confused. "This was before I had even been twenty minutes in his company," she wrote, "or had an opportunity to do anything to excite his anger." Relations between the two remained cool throughout the trip. "During the whole time, until our return to this city," she wrote, "whatever might have been the superficial show of politeness, I was shown no real consideration or respect."[21] To Barton, Moore's behavior was unforgivable. From that point on, she viewed him as an enemy.

The *Virginia* sailed down the Potomac and into the Chesapeake Bay, halting briefly at Fort Monroe before continuing on to Savannah. It was a "rolling voyage," and Barton soon became ill. Each day she grew weaker. She kept to her berth, but even that didn't help as steam pipes located on the deck above and boilers in the engine room below kept the temperature in her cabin at a sweltering 100 degrees.[22] Not once did Moore stop by to see how she was feeling. His lack of common courtesy puzzled and bothered her. "I cannot understand Capt Moore," she confided in her diary. "He does not seem friendly, is silent, and abstract as if I were an intruder, and yet I cannot understand how this can be his feeling as long as the arrangement from the first was mine and not his." Despite his unfriendly behavior, she hoped eventually to win him over with kindness. "How alone I am and on such a trip," she lamented. "How little people at home can realize my situation, and what it will *cost* me."[23]

The *Virginia* reached Savannah on July 12. From there, Moore planned to transport his party to Andersonville by rail. The four-hundred-mile route would pass through the cities of Augusta, Atlanta, and Macon. Upon reaching Savannah, however, he learned that the line was out of order between Savannah and Augusta. He informed members of the party that the expedition might have to turn back.[24] Barton was not about to let that happen. When she went ashore at Savannah on July 14, an army clerk told her that shallow-draft steamships could carry her party up the Savannah River as far as Augusta, bypassing the break in the line. Rather than inform Moore of this privately, Barton made it a point to publicly refute Moore's assertion that they could not go forward. She did so at a dinner party that both of them attended, adding that she had positive information that they could reach Augusta by ship. When Moore still hesitated to advance, it confirmed Barton's suspicions that he wanted the expedition to fail. What she apparently did not know was that the rail line was broken in *two* places, between Savannah and Augusta and again between Augusta and Macon. When, after a week of waiting, Moore finally received word that construction crews had repaired the rail line beyond Augusta, he ordered the expedition to proceed. Nevertheless, Barton continued to think ill of her nemesis, insisting that he had continued forward only because Quartermaster General Montgomery Meigs had ordered him to do so.[25]

The party started upriver on July 19. The working party sailed aboard the transport *Augusta*, while Moore, Atwater, and Barton followed with the supplies aboard the freight ship *Hellen*.[26] Still smarting from Barton's public rebuke a few days earlier, Moore did not offer to escort her to the ship, forcing her to get a ride with a friend instead. "If I had not done so I should have been left," she complained, "as no one was to call on me. Capt Moore told Capt Starr that the boat would go at the precise hour whether I was there or not."[27] Obviously, Moore had not forgotten about Barton's tardy arrival back in Washington.

The trip up the Savannah River was almost as bad as the trip down the Atlantic coast had been. Being a freighter, the ship had no accommodations for passengers, compelling Barton to sleep on a mattress placed on the deck. To make matters worse, a group of Catholic girls was traveling on board the same ship, and they were up all night constantly stepping over her.[28] Fortunately, the trip aboard the *Hellen* lasted just two days. On July 21, Barton, Moore, and Atwater transferred to the *Augusta*, a more comfortable ship offering private cabins. Moore continued to avoid his female associate. "I scarce see Capt. Moore once a day," Barton complained. "He does not wait for me to answer the bell for my meals always, but walks in without me." Rather than suffering the indignity of going to the dining room alone, Barton simply went without dinner. She later recalled that Moore attempted to excuse his rudeness by "professing to be *distracted* with business every minute and vexed to death with poor transportation and slack quartermasters." She wasn't buying it. Her room aboard the *Augusta* offered a view of the deck, and she watched while Moore spent hours whiling away the time smoking cigars and chatting with other passengers.[29] He simply did not like her.

Rather than accept that fact and try to make the best of the situation, Barton continued to let Moore's conduct upset her. When the party reached Augusta and Moore did not offer to take her on a drive through the city, she stayed in her hotel room and fumed. She was used to winning men over with her charm and kindness, but with Moore it wasn't working. In the end, she concluded that his animosity toward her sprang from the fact that he was "exasperated at the order to proceed" to Andersonville, "knowing that it suited me." In reality, Moore appears to have resented her simply because she was a woman and therefore, in his view, a nuisance.[30]

While in Augusta, someone attempted to enter Barton's hotel room in the middle of the night. The thief—if that's indeed what it was—turned the key in her lock, but fortunately she had bolted the door from the inside, and he went away. The incident left Barton rattled. She remained awake the rest of the night in fear lest the intruder return. Predictably, she used the incident as a pretext to criticize Moore. "I am all alone," she confided to her diary. "None of the rest of the party near me and Capt Moore does not know what part of the house I am in. I might be killed and buried and he would never know it. I shall not tell him that this attempt was made for he would not care for it." Moore's disdain had clearly become an obsession with her.[31]

On July 23, the party left Augusta and boarded a train for Atlanta, which it found in "terrible condition." It appeared as if Sherman's army had quartered in the city, wrote Barton, "Ay! and fought in it too!" She summed up its condition with a single word: "Shattered."[32] The following day, the group pushed on to Macon. In contrast to Atlanta, Macon had escaped Sherman's vengeance. Although it had a large brick arsenal and armory—both valuable military targets—Barton noted that "its buildings are good and show few marks of the war."[33] She took supper that evening with the district's military commander, Maj. Gen. James H. Wilson, a former general in the Army of the Potomac.[34] The next day, July 25, a train brought her and the rest of the party to Andersonville.[35]

W. A. Griffin met the train at the station. Griffin lived near the prison camp, and after the Confederates had evacuated it he took it upon himself to maintain and enclose the Union cemetery there with the help of twenty former slaves. When Wilson learned of his activities, he appointed Griffin temporary superintendent over the cemetery and provided rations for both him and his workers.[36] Thanks to Griffin's efforts, Barton found the cemetery in much better order than she anticipated. "I find that the graves can be identified perfectly," she exalted, "my plan is practical again."[37] Moore and his work crew arrived later in the day and began setting up camp a few hundred yards outside the prison walls.[38] In the meantime, Barton took temporary quarters in Griffin's house.[39]

Barton found the prison camp and its structures "almost precisely in the condition in which they had been evacuated."[40] "Nothing has been disturbed," she wrote an acquaintance, "the entire stockade is standing, and . . . the burial grounds have been preserved from everything like desecration, and must have been even *improved* in appearance."[41] The camp looked as if the occupants had just departed. With the exception of Griffin and his crew, thought Barton, "we appear to have been the first upon this saddened spot since the departure of the prisoners and the flight of the frightened guard. Everything about the forts denote[s] a hasty exist."[42] The camp, she learned, had originally encompassed nineteen acres, but as the number of prisoners swelled it had been enlarged to more than twenty-seven acres.[43] Built in the shape of a rectangle, it stood in the middle of what once had been a pine forest.[44] A small stream made "foul and loathesome" by human waste from a Confederate camp upstream constituted the compound's primary source of water, although prisoners had dug as many as forty wells in an effort to augment the supply. There were no barracks. To shelter themselves from the elements, prisoners had either crowded into tents or burrowed like rabbits into the slopes of the undulating ground.[45]

Surrounding the camp were two concentric palisades and an incomplete portion of a third. A "dead line" located approximately eighteen feet inside the inner wall marked the point beyond which prisoners could not pass. Spaced at thirty-yard intervals along the top of the inner palisade were fifty-two sentry boxes in which Confederate soldiers stood guard over the prisoners, while forts armed with field artillery surrounded the camp, discouraging any thought of mass escape. "Truly it looks like the city of the dead," Barton reflected, and indeed it was. Inside this small but strongly guarded enclosure as many as forty-five thousand Union soldiers had

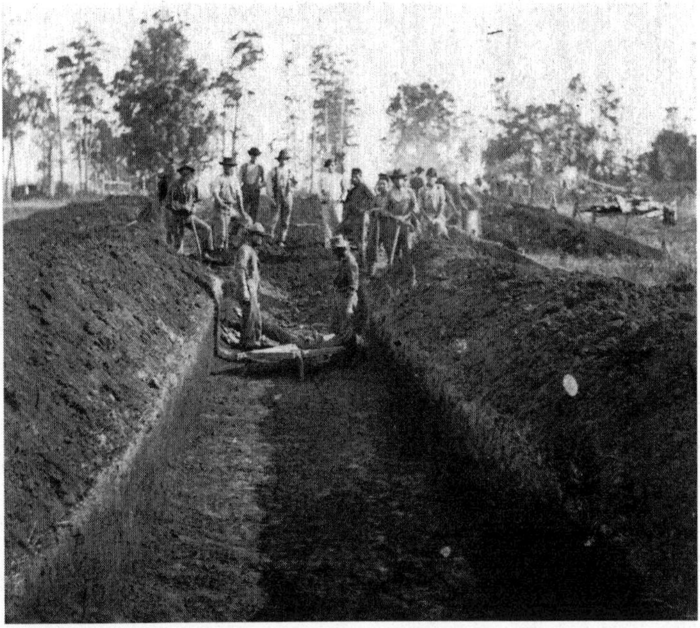

Prisoners burying the dead in a trench at Andersonville Prison, photographed by Andrew J. Riddle. (*Library of Congress*)

been imprisoned during the camp's fourteen-month history. Thirteen thousand of them had died and been buried in a twenty-seven-acre cemetery located three hundred yards northwest of the stockade. That was the ground that Moore had come to preserve and mark.[46]

Work on the cemetery started on July 26. The workers began by completing the fence that Griffin was building around the property and by deepening the shallow graves. They then inscribed and erected six thousand white headboards over the graves, laid out walkways, placed appropriate signs at the gates and along the avenues, and erected a flagstaff in the center of the grounds. Thanks to Atwater's register, Moore was able to identify and mark all but 451 of the plots. Those he could not identify received a headboard that read simply "Unknown U.S. Soldier."[47]

Barton engaged in none of this. From the start Moore had "systematically ignored" her, and now that she was at the prison she realized "that I was not to be consulted about anything, shown anything, or informed of anything that was done, or in contemplation. . . . My opinion was never asked on any question of taste or fitness," she later informed Stanton. "No word of consultation ever passed between Captain Moore and myself, and so forcibly was I impressed from the first by his silence, that I was never once betrayed into making an inquiry or a suggestion." During the three weeks she was at Andersonville, Moore never once asked her to visit the cemetery.[48]

Having been excluded from the practical work of establishing the cemetery, Barton kept herself busy entertaining callers, writing letters, and nursing the sick. Local residents flocked to the cemetery shortly after the work crew's arrival, curious as to what was going on. A group of white ladies, hearing that a Northern woman was in the party, stopped by Barton's tent to pay her a visit. They freely admitted that Union prisoners had received cruel treatment, but protested that, as civilians, they had been powerless to do anything about it.[49]

Most of Barton's visitors placed responsibility for the horrid conditions squarely on the shoulders of Capt. Henry Wirz, the prison commandant, a man with a reputation for intimidation, cruelty—even murder.[50] Barton seethed as local residents related to her stories of Wirz's inhuman treatment of the Andersonville prisoners. "If their reports are *true*," she wrote, "he would have been a '*Star*' in the days of the Spanish Inquisitions."[51] So notorious were Wirz's crimes that after the war he was brought before a military tribunal and charged with murder and conspiracy to kill or injure prisoners. Barton wanted to be a witness at his trial, but her testimony was not required.[52] In the end, Wirz was found guilty of eleven counts of murder and was sent to the gallows on November 10, 1865, one of only two men executed for crimes committed during the war.[53]

Barton's most welcome visitor while at Andersonville was Col. Joel R. Griffin, W. A. Griffin's brother, who was an agent in the employment of the United States Government.[54] As former commander of the 62nd Georgia Mounted Infantry, Colonel Griffin had spent much of the war along the Chowan River in northeastern North Carolina, where he had met and become friends with Barton's older brother, Stephen.[55] The colonel's appearance at Andersonville at a time when she had few other friends struck Barton as nothing short of providential. "How can this thing [have] happened?" she wondered. "Who has directed? Does poor old brother Ste[phen] look down on this cemetery and smile that sweet smile of love and satisfaction that sat so often upon his noble face? I cannot help thinking or *feeling* so, and here beside me tonight has sat the same Col Griffin that used to sit by him and cheer the lonely weary hours of his heartbreaking exile, and here in all this desolation in this strange spot, the last in creation I [could expect] this meeting. . . . Am I crazy? but both God and [my] brother seem very near tonight."[56] Over the next two weeks, Griffin made frequent calls on Barton, inviting her to his home, taking rides with her around the camp, and even helping her draft official letters. He was her friend at a time when she badly needed a one.[57]

Far greater in number than the white residents who came to see Barton were the hundreds of former slaves who visited her. They came from as far as twenty miles away, bringing gifts of food such as chickens, tomatoes, peaches, and milk. Some wished to sell her their produce. Although Barton did not need the food, she usually bought some anyway, "largely as I do not like to have them disappointed," she explained.[58] While many came simply because they were curious to see a Yankee woman, others, remembered Barton, came to "lay their troubles before me and ask my advice."[59] Some were worried because the white people had told them that President Lincoln was dead and that consequently they were no longer free. Others had been run off the land by their former owners or had been denied their wages and wanted to know what they could do about it. Barton advised them as she thought best.[60]

She also managed to do some nursing while at Andersonville.[61] In one instance, she spent the night at the house of a local resident caring for a child suffering from colic.[62] At other times, she kept vigil at the bedside of Edward Watts, a member of the work party who was afflicted with typhoid fever. Barton considered Watts "a young man of education and refinement, and of the highest type of moral and religious character," and took a keen interest in his welfare.[63] She read the Bible to him, made him custard and tea, and changed the linens on his cot. When she could not tend to him herself, she

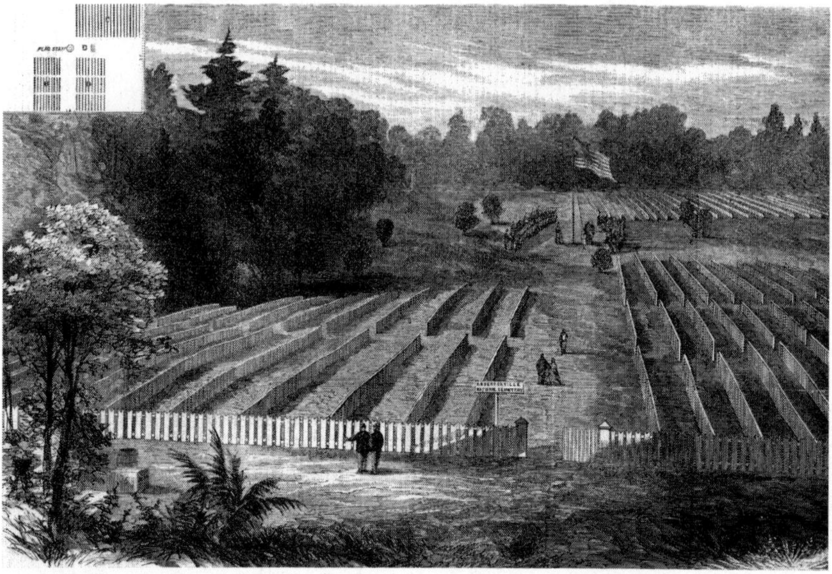

Clara Barton raises the U.S. flag at Andersonville. (*Harper's Weekly*)

hired a black woman to take her place.[64] But despite her efforts Watts grew weaker each day. It was clear he was not going to recover. As death approached, Barton and Atwater took turns sitting up with him throughout the night.[65] Their vigil ended with his death early on August 15. In his final hours, Watts raised his "poor white cold hands" and prayed aloud to his mother in heaven, while Atwater wept at his side. Both men had lost their parents early in life. "I was overcome by the solemnity of the scene," wrote Barton, "there in that little moonlighted tent those two poor orphan boys, weeping for their mothers gone to heaven and left them, one on the verge of the grave and the other just escaped it." She took Watts's hands and found them "cold & clammy." While Atwater rubbed them with a flannel cloth to increase their circulation, Barton wrapped the patient's feet in a white blanket. Piteously, Watts asked Barton if he might "go home." Barton said that he might. A short time later, he spoke again: "Miss Barton is it almost time for me to go home?" "Almost," she replied. After that, his breathing became shorter. Eventually it stopped altogether.

"My God," exclaimed Atwater, "he is dead."

"Yes," replied Barton.

Atwater knelt beside Watts, sobbing. Barton quietly took a place at his side, and together they invoked God's blessing on their deceased friend. At length, Atwater rose, emotionally spent. "He is with his mother now," he said.[66] "Thus went out the christian life of the *last martyr* of Andersonville," wrote Barton. "Few died better or more nobly."[67]

Watts died just as work on the cemetery was coming to an end. In a belated nod toward reconciliation, Moore invited Barton to help raise the United States flag over the cemetery at its August 17 dedication. "I advanced to the side of Mr. Walker, and together we ran it up amid the cheers of the beholders," she recalled. "Up, and there it drooped as if in grief & sadness, till at length, the sunlight streamed out and its beautiful folds filled. The men struck up the Star Spangled Banner and I covered my face and wept. Three volleys—the Red White & blue—and we turned towards our camp and breakfast. The work was done!"[68]

Hours later, Barton was on a train heading back to Washington. With her went Moore and Atwater. Their route took them through Atlanta, Chattanooga, and Nashville—scenes of some of the heaviest fighting of the war. On August 22, they reached Cincinnati, Ohio. Earlier in the month, the *Cincinnati Daily Commercial* and other newspapers had published two letters purportedly written by Barton from Andersonville that briefly described the progress of Moore's party.[69] The articles made it appear that Barton was in charge of the expedition and that Moore was under her authority. Barton denounced the letters as forgeries, insisting they made her appear "odious" and "ridiculous." She privately believed that Moore was the author, although she couldn't prove it. Moore denied having anything to do with the letters, although he did seem to enjoy the annoyance they caused his companion.[70] In an effort to get under her skin, he asked Barton laughingly "if some *friend* of mine [had] not published some letter I had written." Barton replied sharply that she "claimed for myself & friends both common honesty & common sense. It might be the work of either his or my enemy," she asserted, "but not of my friends."[71] That evening, after Maj. Gen. Grenville Dodge boarded the train, Moore brought up the topic of the forged letters again, jokingly telling Dodge that he was under Barton's command. Barton bristled at the comment and "asked Cap M. in the Genls presence if he had been unduly directed or ordered or interfered with by me." According to Barton, Moore "replied that he was ready to affirm both in public and private that he had not been."[72] The incident only served to sharpen Barton's resentment toward her antagonist. Upon reaching Washington on August 24, she sent a report of the expedition to Secretary Stanton, much of which was devoted to vilifying Moore.[73]

Time did not soften Barton's feelings. Four months after the expedition, when reflecting on the events of that year, she wrote: "In only one instance have I met malignity or intentional injury. this although I can forgive, I cannot forget and perhaps it is not desirable or advisable that I should as my enemy is still abroad, and I have him to avoid, and guard against. I allude to the assumed leader of the Expedition to Andersonville. I shall not attempt to oppose him more, but unless I have made a very erroneous estimate of his motives, and the nature of the acts he has perpetrated, I believe he has got some difficulties to meet and overcome which will try both his manhood and strength. I leave him with his God."[74] Barton's animosity toward Moore did nothing to hinder his career. Before the year ended, the army awarded him a brevet promotion to lieutenant colonel for his "faithful and meritorious service" to the country.[75]

Barton's bitterness toward Moore stemmed not only from his behavior toward her during the Andersonville expedition but also from his treatment of Dorence Atwater after their return. While at Andersonville, Atwater had had access to the death register he had copied during the war. Once he returned to Washington, however, his superior in the Quartermaster Department demanded that he either return the document or refund the $300 that the government had paid him for it. Atwater refused to do either, maintaining that he had only loaned his register to government officials so that they could make a copy of it. The original document, he asserted, belonged to him. Atwater's superior responded by placing him under arrest for theft. In short order, he was hauled before a court-martial, convicted, and sentenced to eighteen months of hard labor. Barton blamed Atwater's imprisonment on Moore, who worked in the

Quartermaster Department and apparently countenanced his arrest. "He has accomplished his purposes now with Dorr," she wrote of Moore in the wake of Atwater's conviction, "and now is working quietly upon me I suspect." Ironically, when first arrested, Atwater was confined in Washington's Old Capitol Prison, the same place where Henry Wirz was being held. Subsequently moved to Auburn State Prison in New York, Atwater was released after just two months by order of President Andrew Johnson.[76]

Barton had worked quietly behind the scenes in an effort to secure Atwater's release, and now that he was free she employed him as a clerk at the Missing Soldiers Office.[77] She was able to pay him a salary thanks to a bill passed by Congress in March 1866 granting her $15,000: $12,000 to reimburse her for expenses she had incurred on behalf of wounded soldiers during the war and $3,000 more to further the work of the Missing Soldiers Office. The idea originated with Barton and was pushed through Congress by Wilson.[78] It would be interesting to know how she justified the $12,000 figure. With the Quartermaster Corps providing her wartime transportation and Northern citizens supplying most of the goods she distributed among the soldiers, it's hard to imagine that she spent even $1,200 of her own funds, much less $12,000.[79] It's doubtful Barton even had that much money. She had been strapped for cash throughout the war, her only income during that period being the $25 half salary she got each month from the Patent Office, money that she continued to receive despite no longer working there. In 1865, even that meager income disappeared when a new secretary of the interior eliminated her position. The financial hardship caused by her loss of wages may have been the impetus for her petitioning Congress for funds.[80]

POSTWAR ENDEAVORS

Even before receiving the congressional appropriation, Barton was looking at ways to raise funds for herself and the Missing Soldiers Office. At the urging of her mentor and friend Frances Gage, she decided to try her hand at public speaking. "I have for a long time been quite disheartened," she confided to her diary, "but with the commencement of the new year, I have commenced a new life, determined to follow closely my own purposes, strive to accomplish something for myself; Accordingly I have closed my doors upon all, and set down to write some lectures for reading in public."[81] Starting in 1866 she began giving speeches about her wartime experiences to audiences throughout the North and Midwest. Citizens in towns such as Bloomington, Illinois; Norwalk, Ohio; and Oshkosh, Wisconsin, paid between twenty-five and fifty cents apiece to hear Barton describe her efforts to bring aid and comfort to the wounded. Her tales of suffering, told in a "low, sweet voice," brought tears to the eyes of her listeners, who lavished her with ovations and praised her devotion to the Union. As she traveled from town to town, her fame increased. So did her bank balance. In one month alone she delivered no fewer than twenty-two lectures, each of which brought in between $75 and $100—this at a time when the average salary in the United States was $28.54 per month. The lectures did more than simply provide Barton with a measure of financial independence; they gave her the public attention and recognition she so desperately craved. Just as important, they provided her with a public forum in which to drum up support for three causes she held dear to her heart: Dorence Atwater, the Missing Soldiers Office, and impoverished, wounded Union veterans.[82]

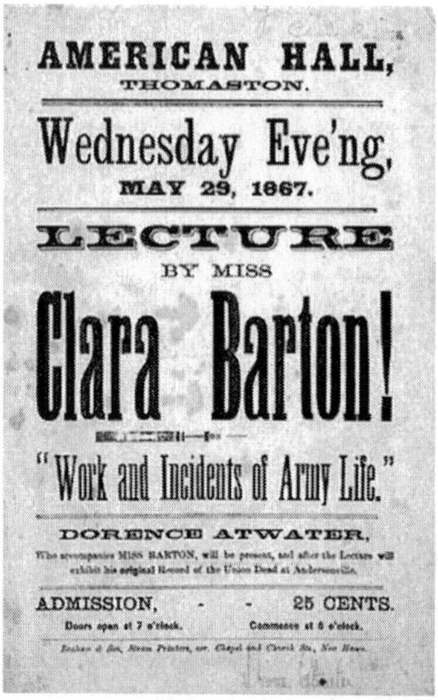

Poster advertising a Barton lecture. (*Plymouth Historical Society, Plymouth, Connecticut*)

The constant travel required to make these public appearances took its toll. In 1868, Barton became so ill that she had to cancel her engagements and go to Europe to recover her health. She was living in Switzerland two years later when the Franco-Prussian War began. Volunteering her services to the International Red Cross, which was aiding victims of that war, she set off for the front. She never made it. Forbidden by military authorities to pass through their lines, she had to abandon the venture and return to Switzerland, having

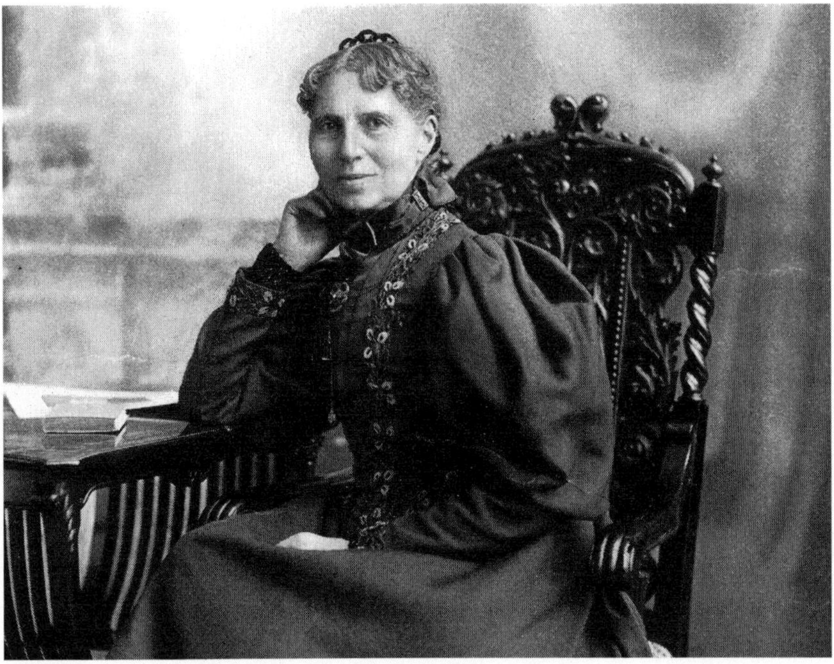

Clara Barton, c. 1910. (*Library of Congress*)

accomplished nothing. Nevertheless, she later claimed to have reached the front and done service there. "It is difficult to know just why Barton consistently exaggerated her hardships and accomplishments," wrote one of her biographers. "Certainly the truth would have brought strong enough accolades." Yet, as in the Civil War, she felt it necessary to amplify her deeds.[83]

Barton returned to the United States in 1873. Following her return, she suffered a nervous breakdown and spent two years recovering in a sanitarium. She gradually improved and by 1877 was seeking new fields of endeavor. With the approval of officials at the International Red Cross headquarters in Switzerland, she set out to persuade the U.S. government to sign the Geneva Treaty, an international accord regulating the treatment of wounded and captured soldiers. Her efforts culminated with U.S. ratification of the treaty in 1882.[84] At the same time, she organized the American chapter of the International Red Cross. As its first president, Barton garnered favorable publicity for the organization and gave it direction. The chapter helped thousands of people during her twenty-three years at the helm, responding effectively to victims of floods, hurricanes, wars, and epidemics. "My work was, and chiefly has been to get timely supplies to those needing [them]," she later explained. "It has taught me the value of 'Things.'" For her efforts in what she called "the paths of charity," Barton received accolades both at home and abroad, including medals from European royalty. By the time she retired from public service in 1904, at the age of eighty, she had become one of America's best known and most beloved public figures.[85]

Still it was not enough. Although lauded as a national heroine, she remained the same painfully insecure individual she had been as a child. When she was invited to attend a reunion of the 21st Massachusetts, a newspaper correspondent reported that she stepped to the platform "amidst loud applause, and, dipping the loose wrap from her shoulders, displayed her breast covered with decorations bestowed upon her by foreign governments as well as by those of her own countrymen. The whole audience, rising, gave three rousing cheers."[86] To the end of her days, she carried her medals around with her like an emotional safety blanket. Neighbors who lived near Barton's Glen Echo, Maryland, home often saw the aged humanitarian working quietly in her yard, the emblems dangling from her calico dress. Although her days of glory had passed, she could not let them go.[87]

Clara Barton died of chronic pneumonia on April 12, 1912, at the age of ninety. A grateful nation buried her near her childhood home in North Oxford, Massachusetts, where her grave can still be seen today.[88] As word of her death spread, newspapers throughout the country joined in praising her for her sacrifice and compassion. "Clara Barton was more than brave," wrote one. "She was one of the most useful women, self-sacrificing to a degree, generous to a fault. Health and fortune she devoted to her great cause. . . . Into the span of what other life have more mercy, tenderness and love entered?"[89] The editor of *The Outlook* magazine added, "It is understating the fact to say that through Clara Barton's initiative, encouragement, and example many thousands of destitute and

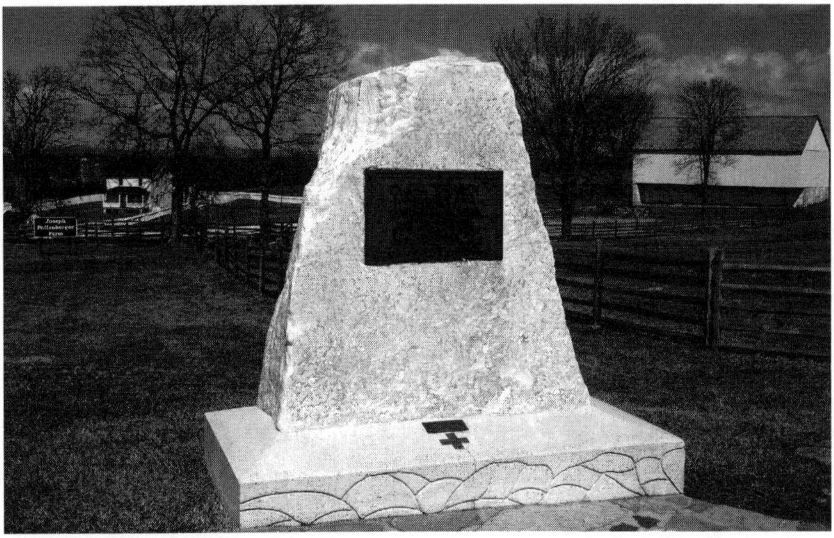

Clara Barton Monument at Antietam National Battlefield. (*Author*)

suffering people have been helped and comforted. Her deeds lend honor to her country's name."[90]

Clara Barton deserved the encomiums she received. Humane and energetic, she had dedicated her life to helping others and in doing so had saved or improved the lives of countless Americans. Although she often exaggerated her accomplishments, she nevertheless merits praise both as a Civil War nurse and for her later work in disaster relief. Since her death, she has been honored in a number of ways. In addition to the many books and articles written about her, she has a plaque in the nation's capital, monuments at Antietam and Andersonville, and a sign in Fredericksburg noting her accomplishments. Dansville, New York, where she once owned a country house, holds a festival each year in her honor, and no fewer than three historic buildings where she lived and worked have been preserved and are now open to the public.[91] If that was not enough, at least one high school and a dozen elementary schools have been named after her, not to mention a cemetery, a community center, and a library. Even a rest stop on the New Jersey Turnpike and a giant sequoia tree in California bear her name. Barton would be pleased. Throughout her life she desperately sought public recognition and praise. She would be gratified to know that, more than a hundred years after her death, Americans still honor her memory.

Appendix

CLARA BARTON IN HER OWN WORDS

Nothing conveys the personality of an historical figure so much as reading his or her own words. A person's writing provides a window into their soul. Diaries and private correspondence are the best guides, for they are written without restraint. Articles, speeches, and other monographs written for public consumption may be less honest, but even they can tell us a great deal about those who wrote them.

Much of what we know about Clara Barton's activities in the Civil War comes from two speeches that she delivered to audiences throughout the North in the years immediately following the Civil War. The excerpts from the first speech that appears here cover Barton's experiences at Fairfax Station, South Mountain, and Antietam. The speech goes by the name that Barton herself gave to it: "Work and Incidents of Army Life." The second speech that follows covers Barton's activities at Fredericksburg, where she served in December 1862 and again in May 1864. She did not assign a name to that speech, and it is sometimes referred to simply as the Black Book.

Like many nineteenth-century writers, Barton's spelling and punctuation were erratic—at least by the precise standards of the present age. Sentences might end in a period, a dash, a semicolon, or any combination thereof. Dashes often took the place of commas, and they often appeared at the beginning or end of a sentence for no apparent reason except that the writer felt that they belonged there. Many writers, including Barton, regarded capitalization at the beginning of a sentence as optional. Such anomalies interfere with the reader's understanding of the text. For that reason, I have chosen to keep Barton's words but to change her punctuation, spelling, and capitalization so as to bring them more closely into line with modern standards. This in no way impairs the meaning of her words; indeed, it makes them clearer.

Here, then, is Clara Barton's story as she herself wrote it.

EXCERPTS FROM "WORK AND INCIDENTS OF ARMY LIFE": FAIRFAX STATION, SOUTH MOUNTAIN, AND ANTIETAM

Let me pass on without comment over the first year [of the war], commencing with the battle of 2d Bull Run and the wounded of Fairfax Station, which point I sought by rail the day after the defeat of General Pope. I had just returned from the battle of Cedar Mountain, where we labored five days without sleep or food (worthy of the name), barely escaped capture, and were gathering the wounded in hospitals at Washington when on Saturday afternoon word came that General Pope was fighting on the Old Bull Run battle ground, had 8000 killed and the battle still went on.[1] That night was spent in packing supplies, which at daybreak in the midst of a heavy rain were placed in freight cars, and with two ladies and my attendants I found a place to stand among the boxes while we steamed and rattled out of Washington. Our coaches were not elegant or commodious: they had no seats, no windows, no platforms, no steps. A slide door on the side was the only entrance and this higher than my head. For my manner of attaining my elevated position, I must beg of you to draw upon your own imaginations and spare me the labor of reproducing the boxes, barrels, boards, and rail, which in those days, seemed to help me up and on in the world. We did not criticize the unsightly helpers and were only too thankful that the stiff springs and siding track did not quite jostle us out at the door on the opposite side. This description need not be limited to this particular trip or train but will suffice for all that I have known in Army life. This is the kind of conveyance by which your tons of generous gifts have reached the field with this [*sic*] precious freights. These trains, through day and night, sunshine and rain, heat and cold have thundered on over heights, across plains, through ravines, and over hastily built army bridges 90 feet above the rocky stream beneath.

At 10 o'clock Sunday our long train drew up at Fairfax Station. The rainy morning had grown to a misty drizzling day, unpleasant with the best of surroundings, and in ten minutes our barrels and boxes of supplies were unloaded and ranged along the track. The ground for acres was a thinly wooded slope, and among the trees on the leaves and grass were laid the wounded who were pouring in by scores of wagon loads as picked up on the field under flag of truce. All day they came and the whole hillside was covered. Bales of hay were broken up and scattered over the ground like litterings for cattle, and the sore, famishing men were laid upon it, and when night shut down in mist and darkness about us we knew that standing apart from the world of anxious, stricken hearts throbbing over the whole country we were a little band of almost empty-handed workers, literally by ourselves in the wild woods of Virginia with 3000 suffering, dying men crowded upon the few acres within our reach.

After gathering up every available implement of convenience for our work, our domestic inventory stood: 2 Water-buckets, 5 tin cups, 1 camp kettle, 1 stew pan, 2 lanterns, 4 bread knives, 3 plates, and [a] 2 quart tin dish—and 3000 guests to serve. You will perceive by this that I had not yet learned to equip myself, for I was not Pallas ready armed but grew into my work by hard thinking and sad experience. It may possibly serve to relieve your momentary apprehension for the future of my labors if I assure you that I was never caught so again, for later I became a notable housekeeper, if that might be said of one who had no house to keep but lived in fields and woods and tents and wagons with all out of doors for a cooking range, mother earth for a kitchen hearth, and the winds of Heaven for a chimney.

You have read of adverse winds. To realize this term in its fullest sense you have only to build a campfire and attempt to cook something by it. There is not a soldier within the sound of my voice but will sustain me in the assertion that, go whichsoever side of it you will, the wind will blow the smoke and flame directly in your face.

Notwithstanding these difficulties, within fifteen minutes from the time of our arrival we were preparing food and dressing wounds. You wonder what and how prepared and how administered without dishes. You generous, thoughtful mothers and wives have not forgotten the tons of preserves and fruits with which you filled our hands. Huge boxes of these stood beside that railway track. Every can, jar, bucket, bowl, cup, or tumbler, when emptied, that instant became a vehicle of mercy to convey some preparation of mingled bread and wine or soup or coffee to some helpless, famishing sufferer who partook of it with the tears rolling down his bronzed cheeks and divided his blessings between the hands that fed him and his god.

I never realized until that day how little a human being could be grateful for, and that day's experience also taught me the utter worthlessness of that which could not be made to contribute directly to our necessities. Of what real value was that which could not save life? The bit of bread which would rest on the surface of a gold eagle was worth more than the coin itself.

But the most fearful scene was reserved for the night. I have said that the ground was littered with dry hay and that we had only two lanterns, but there was plenty of candles. The wounded were laid so close that it was impossible to move about in the dark. The slightest misstep brought a torrent of groans from some poor mangled fellow in your path. Consequently, here were scenes of persons of all grades from the careful man of god, who walked with a prayer upon his lips, to the careless driver hunting for his lost whip, each wandering about among this hay with an open, flaming candle in his hand. The slightest accident, the mere dropping of a light, would have enveloped in flames this whole mass of helpless men.

How we watched and pleaded and cautioned as we worked and wept that night. How we put socks and slippers upon their cold damp feet, wrapped your blankets and quilts about them, and [when] we had no longer these to give, how we covered them in the hay and left them to their rest.

The slight, naked chest of a fair-haired lad caught my eye and, dropping down beside him, I bent low to draw the remnant of his torn blouse about him when, with a quick cry, he threw his left arm across my neck and burying his face in the folds of my dress wept like a child at his mother's knee. I took his poor distressed head in my hands and held it until his great burst of grief should pass away. "And you do not know me?" he said at length. "I am Charley Hamilton, who used to carry your satchel home from school." My faithful pupil, poor Charley, that mangled right arm will never carry a satchel again.[2]

About 3 o'clock in the morning I observed a surgeon with his little flickering candle in hand approaching me with cautious step far up in the wood. "Lady," he said as he drew near, "will you go with me? Out on the hills is a poor distressed lad, mortally wounded and dying. His piteous cries for his sister have touched all our hearts and none of us can relieve but rather seem to distress him by our presence."

By this time I was following him back over his bloody track with great beseeching eyes of anguish on every side looking up in our faces saying so plainly "Don't step on us."

"He can't last half an hour longer," said the surgeon as we toiled on. "He is already quite cold—shot through the abdomen—a terrible wound." By this time, his cries became greatly audible to me.

"Mary! Mary! Sister Mary! Come, oh, come! I am wounded Mary. I am shot. I am dying. Oh, come to me. I have called you so long and my strength is almost gone. Don't let me die here alone. Oh, Mary, Mary come!"

Of all tones of entreaty to which I have ever listened—and certainly I have had some experience of sorrow—I think these, sounding through that dismal night, the most heartrending. As we drew near some twenty persons, attracted by his cries, had gathered around and stood with moistened eyes and helpless hands waiting the change which would relieve them all, and in the[ir] midst, stretched upon the ground, lay a scarcely full-grown young man with a graceful head of hair, tangled and matted, thrown back from a forehead and a face of livid whiteness. His throat was bare; his hands, bloody red, clasped above his breast; his large, bewildered blue eyes turning anxiously in every direction, and ever from between his ashen lips pealed that piteous cry of "Mary, Mary, come." I approached him unobserved and, motioning the lights away, I knelt by him alone in the darkness. Shall I confess that I intended, if possible, to cheat him out of his terrible death agony? But my lips were truer than my heart and would not speak the word "brother" I had willed them to do. So I placed my hands upon his neck, kissed his cold forehead, and laid my cheek against his.

The illusion was complete; the act had done the falsehood my lips refused to speak. I can never forget that cry of joy, "Oh Mary! Mary! have you come? I knew you would come if I called you, and I have called you so long. I could not die without Mary. Don't cry darling. I'm not afraid to die, and you came to me. Oh bless you! Bless you, Mary!" and he ran his cold, blood-wet hands about my neck, passed them over my face, and twined them in my hair, which by this time had freed itself from fastenings and was hanging damp and heavy upon my shoulders. He gathered the loose locks in his stiffened fingers and holding them to his lips continued to whisper through them. "Bless you, bless you, Mary!" And I felt the hot tears of joy trickling from the eyes I had thought stony in death. This encouraged me and, wrapping his feet closely in blankets and giving him such stimulants as he could take, I seated me on the ground and lifted him on my lap and drawing the shawl on my own shoulders also about his I bade him rest. I listened till his blessings grew fainter, and in ten minutes with them upon his lips he fell asleep.

So the gray morning found us. My precious charge had grown warm and was comfortable. Of course, the morning light would reveal his mistake, but he had grown calm and was refreshed and able to endure it, and when finally he awoke, he seemed puzzled for a moment and smiling said, "I knew before I opened my eyes that this couldn't be Mary. I know now that she couldn't get here, but it is almost as good. You've made me so happy."

"Who is it?" I said it was simply a lady who, hearing that he was wounded, had come to care for him. He wanted the name and with childlike simplicity spelled it letter by letter to know if he were right. "In my pocket," he said, "you will find mother's last letter. Please get it and write your name upon it, for . . . for I want both names by me when I die."

"Will they take away the wounded?" he asked.

"Yes," I replied. "The first train for Washington is nearly ready now."

"I must go," he said quickly.

"Are you able?" I asked.

"I must go if I die on the way. I'll tell you why. I am poor mother's only son, and when she consented that I should come to the war I promised her faithfully that if I were not killed outright, but wounded, I would try every means in my power to be taken home to her, dead or alive. If I die on the train they will not throw me off, and if buried in Washington she can get me, but out here in the Virginia woods in the hands of the enemy—never. I must go."

I sent for the surgeon in charge of the train and requested that my boy be taken.

"Oh, impossible madam. He is mortally wounded and will never reach a hospital. We must take those who have a hope of life."

"But you must take him."

"I cannot."

"Can you, Doctor, guarantee the lives of all you have on that train?"

"I wish I could," said he sadly. "They are the worst cases. Nearly fifty per cent must die eventually of their wounds and hardships."

"Then give this lad his chance with them. He can only die and he has given good and sufficient reasons why he must go, and a woman's word for it, Doctor, you take him. Send your men for him."

Whether yielding to argument or entreaty I neither knew nor cared so long as he did yield, nobly and kindly. And they gathered up the fragments of the poor torn boy and laid him carefully on a blanket in the crowded train, and with stimulants and food and a kind-hearted attendant pledged to take him alive or dead to Armory Square Hospital and tell them he was Hugh Johnson of New York, and to mark his grave, the whistle sounded and the death-freighted train moved on.

Although three hours of my time had been devoted to one sufferer among thousands, it must not be inferred that our general work had been suspended or that my assistants had been equally inefficient. They had seen how I was engaged and nobly redoubled their exertions to make amends for my deficiencies. Probably not a man was laid upon those cars who did not receive some personal attention at their hands, some little kindness, if it were only to help lift him more tenderly, place a pillow or wisp of hay under some broken limb or bruised head, fill his canteen with water, or place a few crackers beside him lest he grow faint on the way. And by these little acts the temper of this entire body of men was changed and [in] the place of complaint and imprecations were only thanks and brave, hopeful assurances that they should get along very well. And as the words of grateful cheer rose up from that moving mass of suffering and doom, I bowed my head in penitence and humbly acknowledged the just rebuke upon all past ingratitude.

This finds us shortly after daylight Monday morning, train after train of cars rushing on for the wounded and scores and hundreds of wagons bringing them in from the field still held by the enemy, where some poor sufferers had lain three days already with no visible means of sustenance. If immediately placed upon the trains and not detained, at least twenty-four hours must elapse before they could be certainly in the hospital and properly nourished. They were already famishing, weak and sinking from loss of blood, and could ill afford a further entire fast of twenty-four hours. I felt confident that, unless nourished at once, all the weaker portion must be past recovery before reaching the hospitals of Washington. If once taken from the wagons and laid with those already cared for, they would be overlooked and perish on the way. Something must be done to meet this fearful emergency. I sought the various officers on the grounds, explained the case to them, and asked permission to feed all the men as they arrived before they should be taken from the wagons. It was well for the poor sufferers of that field that it was controlled by noble-hearted, generous officers, quick to feel and prompt to act. They at once saw the propriety of my request and gave orders that all wagons should be stayed at a certain point and only moved on when everyone had been seen and fed. This point secured, I commenced my day's work of climbing from the wheel to the brake of every wagon, speaking to and feeding with my own hands each soldier until he expressed himself satisfied.

To add to the misery of the scene for me, I encountered among them seven young men who a few years before had been my pupils. [I cannot] impart to you who have never known it—and I would not if I could—the shock and heart-breaking sensation of finding myself suddenly in the presence of a mutilated, perishing human form, which you by no feature recognize, and catch the quick [look] of recognition, and watch the muscles contract and the tears fall, and wait in an agony of suspense for the choking voice to return and tell you who he was in the days when you knew and loved him;—to attempt to recognize in those wan, distorted features, the bright, happy face you were wont to see upturned to your own for counsel and approval:—in that blood-matted hair, the fair locks you have seen parted smoothly from his mother's hand, or tossing in the wind as he shouted at his play, and in that dead, cold hand hanging at his side, waiting the relief of the surgeon's knife and saw, the little boyish fingers your own have taught to trace his name. Imagine seven such scenes crowded into those few hours of confusion and horror, and you have some suggestion of that day's work.[3]

Still there were bright spots along the darkened lines. Early in the morning, the Provost Marshall came to ask me if I could use fifty men. He had that number, who, for some slight breach of military discipline, were under guard and useless—unless I could use them. I only regretted there were not five hundred. They came—strong, willing men—and these, added to our original force and what we had gained incidentally, made our number something over eighty, and believe me eighty men and three women, acting with well directed purpose, will accomplish some work in a day. Our fifty prisoners dug graves and gathered and buried the dead, bore mangled men over the rough ground in their arms, loaded cars, built fires, made soup, and administered it, and I failed to discern that their services were less valuable than those of other men. I had previously suspected, and have since become convinced, that a private soldier may be placed under guard, court-martialed, and even be imprisoned without forfeiting his honor or manliness, that the real dishonor is often upon the Gold Lace rather than the army blue.[4] At three o'clock the last train of wounded left. All day we had known that the enemy hung upon the hills and were waiting to break in upon us, hoping to capture forage, ammunition, and prisoners.

At six o'clock the clouds gathered black and murky, and the low growl of distant thunders ran over our heads, and mingled[5] with the nimble lightnings which illuminated the horizon. The still air grew thick and stifled, and the very branches appeared to droop and bow as if in grief at the memory of the terrible scenes so lately enacted and the gallant lives so nobly yielded up beneath their shelter. This was afternoon of Monday. Since Saturday noon I had not thought of tasting food, and we had just drawn around a box for that purpose when of a sudden! air and earth and all about us shook with one mingled crash of God's and man's artillery. The lightning played and the thunder rolled incessantly, and the cannon roared louder and nearer each minute. Chantilly with all its darkness and horrors had opened in the rear.[6] The description of this battle I leave to those who saw and moved in it, as it is my purpose to speak only of events in which I was a witness or actor. Although two miles distant, we knew the battle was intended for us and watched the firing as it neared and receded and waited minute by minute for the rest.[7]

With what desperation our men fought hour after hour in the rain and darkness. How they were overborne and rallied, how they suffered from mistaken orders and blundered and lost themselves in the strange, mysterious wood, and how after all, with giant strength and veteran bravery, they checked the foe and held him at bay are all proud records of history, and the courage of the soldier who braved death in the darkness of Chantilly let no man question.

> Though in mist and in darkness and fire they were shrouded
> Yet the souls of the righteous were calm and unclouded,
> Their dark eyes flashed lightnings as firm and unbending;
> They stood like the rock that the thunder is rending.[8]

The rain continued to pour in torrents, and the darkness became impenetrable save from the lightning leaping above our heads and the fitful flash of the guns as volley after volley rang through the stifled air and lighted up the gnarled trunks and dripping branches among which we ever waited and listened. In the midst of this—and how guided no man knows—came still another wagon train of wounded men, and a waiting train of cars upon the track received them. This time, nearly alone for my worn-out assistants could work no longer, I continued to administer such food as I had left. Do you begin to wonder what it could be? Army crackers put into knapsacks and haversacks and beaten to crumbs between stones and stirred into a mixture of wine or whiskey and water and sweetened with coarse brown sugar. Not very inviting, you will think, but I assure you always acceptable. But whether it should have been classed as food, or, like the Widow Bedott's Cabbage[9] as "a delightful beverage," it would puzzle an epicure to determine. No matter, so it imparted strength and comfort.

The departure of this train cleared the grounds of wounded for the night, and as the line of fire from its plunging engines died out in the darkness a strange sensation of weakness and weariness fell upon me almost defying my utmost exertion to move one foot before the other. A little Sibley tent[10] had been hastily pitched for me in a slight hollow upon the hillside, but neither ditch or drain of any description. Your imaginations will not fail to picture its condition. Rivulets of water had rushed through it during the last three hours. Still I attempted to reach it, as its white surface, in the darkness, was a slight protection from the wheels of wagons and trampling of beasts.

Perhaps I shall never forget the painful effort which the making of those few rods and the gaining of the tent cost me, how many times I fell from complete exhaustion in the darkness and mud of that slippery hillside. I have no knowledge! But at last I grasped the welcome canvas, and a well established brook which washed in on the upper side and out at the opening that served as door, met me on my entrance. My entire floor was covered with water—not an inch of dry, solid ground.

One of my lady assistants had previously taken train for Washington[11] and the other, worn out by faithful labors, was crouched upon the top of some boxes in one corner, fast asleep. No such convenience remained for me, and I had no strength to arrange one. I sought the highest side of my tent, which I remembered was grass grown, and ascertaining that the water was not very deep, I sank down. It was no laughing matter then, but the recollection of my position has since afforded me amusement. I remember myself sitting on the ground, upheld by my left arm, my head resting on my hand, impelled by an almost uncontrollable desire to lie completely down and prevented by the certain conviction that if I did the water would flow into my ears.

How long I balanced between my desires and cautions I have no positive knowledge, but it is very certain that the former carried the point by the position from which I was aroused at twelve o'clock by the rumbling of more wagons of wounded men. I had slept two hours, and Oh! what strength I had gained! I may never know two other hours of equal worth. I sprang to my feet, dripping wet, covered with ridges of dead grass and leaves, wrung the water from my hair and skirts, and went forth again to my work.

When I stood again under the sky, the rain had ceased. The clouds were sullenly retiring, and the lightning, as if deserted by its boisterous companions, had withdrawn to a distant corner and was playing quietly by itself, for the great volleying thunders of Heaven and Earth had settled down on the fields of Chantilly and the forests of Fairfax—silent. I said so and it was, save the ceaseless rumbling of the never-ending train of army wagons which brought alike the wounded, the dying, and the dead.

And thus the morning of the third day broke upon us—drenched, weary, sore footed, sad hearted, discouraged, and under orders to retreat. A little later, the plaintive wail of a single fife, the slow beat of a muffled drum, the steady tramp, tramp, tramp of heavy feet, the gleam of ten thousand bayonets on the hills, and with bowed heads and speechless lips poor Kearny's leaderless men came marching through. This was the signal for retreat. All day they came: tired, hungry, ragged, defeated, retreating they knew not whither. The enemy's cavalry, skirting the hills, admonished us each moment that we must soon decide to go from them or with them. But our work must be accomplished, and no wounded men once given into our hands must be left, and with the spirit of desperation we struggled on.

At three o'clock, an officer galloped up to me with "Miss Barton, can you ride?"

"Yes Sir," I replied.

"But have you no saddle? Could you ride mine?"

"Yes, or without, if you have blanket or surcingle."[12]

"Then you can risk another hour," he exclaimed and galloped off.

At four o'clock he returned at a breakneck speed and leaping from his horse said, "Now is your time. The cavalry is already breaking over the hills. Try the train. It will go through unless they have flanked and cut the bridge a mile above us. In that case, I have a reserve horse for you, and you must take your chances of escape across the country."

In two minutes I was on the train. The last wounded man at the station was also on. The conductor stood with a torch, which he applied to a pile of combustible material beside the track, and as we rounded the curve which took us from view, we saw the station ablaze and a troop of Rebel Cavalry dashing down the hill. The bridge was uncut and midnight found us at Washington.

You have the full record of my sleep from Friday night till Wednesday morning—two hours. You will not wonder that I slept during the next twenty-four hours. On Friday, I repaired to Armory Square Hospital to learn who of all the hundreds sent had reached that point. I sought the chaplain's record and there upon the last page freshly written stood the name of Hugh Johnson. Turning to Chaplain Jackson, I asked, "Did that man live until today?"

"He died during the latter part of last night," he replied. "His friends reached him some two days ago, and they are now taking his body from the ward to be conveyed to the depot." I looked in the direction his hand indicated, and there beside a coffin about to be lifted into a wagon stood a gentleman, the mother, and sister Mary.

"Had he his reason?" I asked.

"Oh perfectly! And his mother and sister were with him two days!"

Yes, there was no need of me. He had given his own messages; I could add nothing to their knowledge of him and would fain be spared the scene and the thanks. Poor Hugh! Thy piteous prayers reached and were answered, and with eyes and heart full I turned away and never saw sister Mary!

These were days of darkness, a darkness that might be felt. The shattered bands of Pope and Banks, Burnside's weary legions, the men who had followed Frémont over the mountain paths, the reinforcements from West Virginia, and all that now remained of the once glorious army of the Peninsular had gathered for shelter beneath the redoubts and guns that girdled *Washington.*[13] The long maneuvering and skirmishing on the Rappahannock and the Shenandoah had yielded no fruit but this. Gen. Pope's boastful words[14] had turned upon him like causeless curses and all the blood shed from Yorktown to Malvern Hill,[15] seemed to have been utterly in vain. Washington was filled with dismay, and all the North was moved as a tempest stirs a forest.

These however are matters of Public History. But the minor keys upon which I played my infinitesimal notes in the great anthem of war and victory that rang through the land when those two fearful forces met and closed with gunlock kissing gun across the rocky bed of Antietam are yet known only to a few. Who whispered hastily on Saturday night, Oct. 13th, "Harpers Ferry—not a moment to be lost," I have never dared to name. The famishing men of Cedar Mountain and Fairfax had taught me the folly and wickedness of remaining quietly at home until reporters and journalists told us that a battle had been fought and thousands of our men lay dying on the field without food or nursing. I had determined to anticipate trouble and meet it halfway at least.

In thirty minutes I was timidly waiting the always kindly spoken "Come in" of my patron saint Major *now* Maj. General Rucker.[16]

"Major," I said, "I want to go to Harpers Ferry. Can I go?"

He turned upon me the same pleasant smile he always gave me, now uncommonly full of meaning, and replied, "I see no reason why you cannot. Do you want a conveyance?"

"Yes," I said.

"An army wagon is the only vehicle that will reach there with any burden in safety. I will send you one tomorrow morning."

I said I would be ready. I need not tell you that that night brought no sleep. But this was to be a new experience. I was to ride 80 miles in an Army wagon and straight into battle and danger at that. I could take no female companions, even if any desired to accompany me. You who are accustomed to see a coach and pair of fine horses with well dressed gentlemanly drivers draw up to your door will scarcely appreciate the sensation with which I watched the approach of the long, high, white-covered, tortoise-motioned vehicle with its string of little frisky, long-eared animals with the broad-shouldered Dutch driver astride and the eternal jerk of his single rein by which he navigated his craft up to my door. It might [be] proper to state that there has existed a remarkably good understanding between myself and the mule creation during the entire war.

The time you will remember was Sunday, the place 7th St. just off Pennsylvania Avenue, Washington City. Then and there, my vehicle was loaded with boxes, bags, and parcels, and last of all, I found a place to sit down with four men.[17] I took no Saratoga trunk[18] but remembered at the last moment to tie up a few articles in a handkerchief. Thus equipped and seated, my chain of little uneasy animals commenced to straighten itself and soon brought us into the center of Pennsylvania Avenue in full gaze of the inhabitants of the whole city in their best attire and on their way to church. Thus all day we rattled on over the stones and dykes and up and down the hills of Maryland.

At nightfall we turned into an open field and, dismounting, built a campfire, prepared supper, and retired, I to my nook in my wagon, the men wrapped in their blankets about me. All night an indistinct roar of artillery sounded upon our ears. Waking or sleeping, we were conscious of trouble ahead, but it was well for our rest that no messenger came to tell us how death reveled among our brave troops that night.

Before daybreak we had breakfasted and were on our way. You must not infer that because by ourselves we were alone upon the road. We were directly in the midst of a train of army wagons at least ten miles in length moving in solid column, the government supplies of ammunition, food, and medicine for an army in battle. Weary and sick from their late exposures and hardships, the men were failing and falling by the wayside, faint, pale, and often dying. I busied myself as I rode on hour by hour in cutting loaves of bread in slices and passing them to the pale, haggard wrecks as they sat by the roadside or staggered on to avoid capture, and at each little village we entered I purchased all the bread its inhabitants would sell.

Horses as well as men had suffered and their dead bodies strewed the wayside. As we passed on, the residents began to tell us of a great battle fought last night, they said, a few miles up the mountain and that a General was killed. Hastened by anxiety and excitement we were urging on when suddenly we found our wheels crushing the bodies of unburied slain. Unconsciously, and without searching, we had found a battlefield, for this ragged range rising heavily on our right was South Mountain and that fallen General, Reno.[19]

My poor words can never describe to you the consternation and horror with which we descended from our wagon and trod there in that mountain pass that field death. There, where we now walked with peaceful feet, twelve hours before the ground had rocked with carnage. There, in the darkness, God's Angels of wrath and death had swept. And, foe facing foe, freedom and treason grappled and the souls of men went out, and there, side by side, stark and cold in death, mingled the

Northern Blue and Southern Gray. To such of you as have stood in the midst, or followed in the track, of armies and witnessed the strange mingled and dreadful confusion of recent battlegrounds, I need not describe this field, and to you who have not, description would never avail.

The giant rocks hanging above our heads seemed to frown upon the scene, and the sighing trees which hung lovingly upon their rugged edge drooped low and wept their pitying dews upon the livid brows and ghastly wounds beneath. Climbing hills and clambering over ledges we sought in vain for some poor wretch in whom life had still left the power to suffer. Not one remained, and grateful for this but shocked and sick of heart, we returned to our waiting conveyance.

A mammoth drove of cattle designed as rations for our troops was passing at the moment, the officer in charge of which, attracted by our cheerful fire the night previous, had sought our company and been our guest. Scarcely was I seated in my wagon when this officer rode up and said confidently, "Miss Barton, that house on the lower side of the road under the hill has been taken as a Confederate hospital and is full of wounded rebels. Their surgeons have come out and asked me for meat, saying that their men will die for lack of animal food. I am a bonded officer and responsible for the property under my charge. What can I do?"

"You can do nothing," I said, "but ride on ahead. I am neither bonded nor responsible."

He was wise and a word was sufficient. He had a sudden call to the front of his train and dashed forward. Speaking to two of my men, I pointed out a large, white ox slightly strayed from the drove and attempting to graze (He had been with Genl. Pope's army long enough to learn to live off the country) and directed them to drive him to that house inside the fence which surrounded it, put up the bars, and leave him there, asking no questions. I need not say that it was all performed with wonderful alacrity, and the last I saw of the white ox he had gone completely over to the enemy and was reveling in the tall grass about the house. Three years later, as I stood among the 12,000 graves of Andersonville, filled with the skeletons of the martyrs of Freedom, the victims of deliberate starvation, I could not but think how ill that day's generosity had been requited.

Our wounded had been taken on to Fredericktown,[20] where only the day before:

Lee marched over the mountain wall
Over the mountains wandering down
Horse and foot into Fredericktown
Where Old Barba[ra] Frietchie,
Bowed with her fourscore years and ten
Took up the flag and men hauled down
And the staff in her attic window set
To show that one heart was loyal yet.[21]

The increase of stragglers along the road was alarming, showing that our army was weary and lacked not only physical strength but confidence and spirit. And why should they not—always defeated, always on the retreat. I was almost demoralized myself, and I had just commenced.

I have already spoken of the great length of the army train and that we could no more change our position than one of the planets unless we should wait and fall in the rear. We could not advance a single wagon, and for the benefit of those who may not understand, I may explain the order of the train: first, ammunition; next, food and clothing for well troops; and, lastly, hospital supplies. Thus, in case of a battle, the needed stores for the army, according to the slow, cautious movement of such bodies, must be from two to three days in coming up. Meanwhile, as usual, our men must languish and die. Something must be done to gain time, and I resorted to strategy. We found an early resting place, supped by our campfire, and slept again among the dews and damps. At one o'clock, when everything was still, we arose, breakfasted, harnessed, and moved on past the whole train, which, like ourselves, had camped for the night, At daylight, we had gained ten miles and were up with the artillery in advance even of the ammunition.

All that weary, dusty day I followed the cannon, and nightfall brought us up with the great army of the Potomac, 80,000 men resting upon their arms in the face of a foe equal in number—sullen, straightened, and desperate. Closely following the guns, we drew up where they did—among the smoke of a thousand campfires, men hastening to and fro, and the atmosphere loaded with noxious vapors till it seemed the very breath of pestilence. We were upon the left wing of the army, and this was the evening rest of Burnside's men. To how many hundreds it proved the last rest upon earth the next day's record shows.

In all this vast assemblage I saw no other trace of womankind. I was faint but could not eat, weary but could not sleep, depressed but could not weep. So I climbed into my wagon, tied down the cover, dropped down in the little nook I had occupied so long, and prayed God with all the earnestness of my soul to stay the morrow's strife or send us victory; and for my poor self that he impart somewhat of wisdom and strength to my heart, nerve to my arm, speed to my feet, and fill my hands for the terrible duties of the coming day. And heavy and sad I waited its approach.

Many of you may have never heard the bugle notes which call to battle, "The Kerner's breath whose fearful blast would waken death,"[22] but if, like us, you had heard them this morning as they rang through those valleys and echoed from the hundred hills, waking from one sleep to hasten to another, they would have lingered in your ears as they do in mine tonight. With my attendants I sought the hilltops, and as the mist cleared away and the morning sun broke over Maryland Heights, its rays fell upon the dusty forms of 160,000 men, risen like the

> Old Scots from the heather,
> Standing face to face in solemn sullen battle line,
> To hero born for battle strife
> Or bards of martial lay
> Were worth ten years of peaceful life,
> One glance at their array[23]

The battle commenced on the right and already with the aid of field glasses we saw our own forces, though led by fighting Joe,[24] overborne and falling back. Burnside commenced to send cavalry and artillery to his aid and, thinking our place might be there, we followed them around eight miles, turning into a cornfield near a house and barn,[25] and stopping in the rear of the last gun, which completed the terrible line of artillery which ranged diagonally in the rear of Hooker's army that day. A garden wall only separated us. The infantry were already driven back two miles and stood under cover of the guns. The fighting had been fearful. We had met wounded men, walking or borne to the rear for the last two miles, but around the old barn lay there, too badly wounded to admit of removal, some 300 thus early in the day—for it was scarce ten o'clock.

We loosened our mules and commenced our work. The corn was so high as to conceal the house, which stood some distance to the right, but judging that a path which I observed must lead to it and also that surgeons must be operating there, I took my arms full of stimulants and bandages and followed the opening.

Arriving at a little wicker gate, I found the dooryard of a small house and myself face to face with one of the kindest and noblest surgeons I have ever met, Dr. Dunn of Conneautville, Pa. Speechless both, for an instant, he at length threw up his hands with "God has indeed remembered us! How did you get from Virginia here so soon and again to supply our necessities? And they are terrible. We have nothing but our instruments and the little chloroform we brought in our pockets, have torn up the last sheets we could find in this house, have not a bandage, rag, lint, or string, and all these shell-wounded men bleeding to death." Upon the porch stood four tables with an etherized patient upon each, surgeon standing over him with his box of instruments, and a bunch of green corn leaves beside him.[26]

With what joy I laid my precious burden down among them and thought that never before had linen looked so white or wine so red. Oh! Be grateful, ladies, that God put it in your hearts to perform the work you did in those days. How double sanctified was the sacred old household linen woven by the hands of the sainted mother long gone to her reward; for you arose the tender blessings of those grateful men which linger in my memory as faithfully tonight as do the bugle notes which called them to their doom.

Thrice that day was the ground in front of us contested, lost and won, and twice our men were driven back under cover of that fearful range of guns, and each time brought its hundreds of wounded to our crowded ground.

A little after noon the enemy made a desperate attempt to regain what had been lost. Hooker, Sedgwick, Dana, Richardson, Hartsuff and Mansfield had been borne wounded from the field, and the command of the right wing devolved upon General Howard.[27] The smoke became so dense as to obscure our sight, and the hot sulfurous breath of battle dried our tongues and parched our lips to bleeding. We were in a slight hollow and all shell which did not break among our guns, in front, came directly among or over us, bursting above our heads or burying themselves in the hills beyond.

A man lying upon the ground asked for drink. I stooped to give it and, having raised him with my right hand, was holding the cup to his lips with my left when I felt a sudden twitch of the loose sleeve of my dress. The poor fellow sprang from my hands and fell back quivering in the agonies of death. A ball had passed between my body and the right arm which supported him, cutting through the sleeve and passing through his chest from shoulder to shoulder. There was no more to be done for him and I left him to his rest. I have never mended that hole in my sleeve. I wonder if a soldier ever does mend a bullet hole in his coat?

The patient endurance of those men was most astonishing. As many as could be were carried into the barn as a slight protection against random shot. Just outside the door lay a man wounded in the face, the ball having entered the lower maxillary on the left side and lodged among the bones of the right cheek. His imploring look drew me to him. When placing his fingers upon the sharp protuberance, he said, "Lady, will you tell me what this is that burns so?" I replied that it must be the ball, which had been too far spent to cut its way entirely through.

"It is terribly painful," he said, "won't you take it out?" I said I would go to the tables for the surgeon.

"No! No!" he said, catching my dress. "They cannot come to me. I must wait my turn, for this is a little wound. You can get the ball. There is a knife in my pocket. Please take the ball out for me." This was a new call. I had never severed the nerves and fibers of human flesh, and I said I could not hurt him so much. He looked up, with as nearly a smile as such a mangled face could assume, saying, "You cannot hurt me dear lady. I can endure any pain that your hands can create. Please do it. T'will relieve me so much."

I could not withstand his entreaty, and opening the best blade of my pocket knife prepared for the operation. Just at his head lay a stalwart orderly sergeant from Illinois with a face beaming with intelligence and kindness and who had a bullet directly through the fleshy part of both thighs. He had been watching the scene with great interest and when he saw me commence to raise the poor fellow's head, and no one to support it, with a desperate effort he succeeded in raising himself to a sitting posture, exclaiming as he did so, "I will help do that," and shoving himself along upon the ground he took the wounded head in his hands and held it while I extracted the ball and washed and bandaged the face. I do not think a surgeon would have pronounced it a scientific operation, but that it was successful I dared to hope from the gratitude of the patient. I assisted the sergeant to lie down again, brave and cheerful as he had risen, and passed on to others.

Returning in half an hour I found him weeping, the great tears rolling silently down his manly cheeks. I thought his effort had been too great for his strength and expressed my fears. "Oh no! No, Madam," he replied. "It is not for myself; I am very well," but pointing to another just brought in, he said, "This is my comrade and he tells me that our regiment is all cut to pieces, that my captain was the last officer left and he is dead."

Oh! God, what a costly war! This man could laugh at pain, face death without a tremor, and yet weep like a child over the loss of his comrades and his captain.

At two o'clock my men came to tell me that the last loaf of bread had been cut and the last cracker pounded. We had three boxes of wine still unopened. What should they do?

"Open the wine and give that," I said. "And God help us." The next instant an ejaculation from Sergeant Field, who opened the first box, drew my attention, and to my astonished gaze the wine had been packed in nicely sifted Indian meal. If it had been gold dust, it would have seemed poor in comparison. I had no words. No one spoke. In silence, the men wiped their eyes and resumed their work. Of twelve boxes of wine which we carried, the first nine when opened had been found packed in sawdust; the last, when all else was gone, in Indian meal.

A woman would not hesitate long under circumstances like these. This was an old farmhouse. Six large kettles were picked up, washed and filled with water, and set over fires almost as quickly as I can tell it, and I was mixing meal and water for gruel. It occurred to us to explore the cellar. The chimney rested on an arch,[28] and forcing the door we discovered three barrels and a bag. "They are full," said the sergeant as he sounded them with his foot, and rolling one into the light found that it bore the mark of Jackson's army. These three barrels of flour and a bag of salt had been stored by the Rebel Army during its march. I shall never experience such a sensation of wealth and competency again. From utter poverty to such riches!

All that night my thirty men (for our corps of workers had increased to that number during the day) carried buckets of hot gruel for miles down the line to the wounded [and] dying where they fell. This time we had lanterns to hang in and around the barn, and having directed it to be done, I went to the house and found the surgeon in charge sitting alone, beside a table, upon which he rested his elbow apparently meditating upon a tallow candle that flickered in its center. Approaching carefully, I said, "You are tired Doctor."

He started up with a look almost savage. "Tired Yes! I am tired—tired of such heartlessness, such carelessness!" and turning full upon me continued: "Think of the condition of things. Here are at least 1000 wounded men—terribly wounded—500 of whom cannot live till daylight without attention. That two inches of candle is all I have or can get. What can I do? How can I endure it?"

I took him by the arm, and leading him to the door, pointed in the direction of the barn, where the lanterns glistened like stars among the waving corn.

"What is that?" he exclaimed.

"The barn is lighted," I said, "and the house will be directly."

"Who did it?" he asked. "Where did you get them?"

"I brought them with me."

"How many have you?"

"All you want—four boxes."

He looked at me a moment, turned away without a word, and never afterward alluded to the circumstances. But the deference which he paid me was almost painful.

Darkness brought silence and peace, respite and rest to our gallant men, and as they had risen regiment by regiment from their grassy beds in the morning, so at night the fainting remnant again sunk down on the trampled earth, the weary to sleep "and the wounded to die." Through the long, starlit night we wrought and hoped and prayed, but it was only when in the hush of the following day, as we glanced over that vast aceldama,[29] that we learned at what a fearful cost the gallant Union Army won the battle of Antietam.

FREDERICKSBURG 1862 AND 1864

The following text comes from a speech delivered by Clara Barton in the late 1860s describing her experiences in December 1862 during the Battle of Fredericksburg and in May 1864 during the Overland Campaign.[30]

In another lecture I have spoken of Antietam and its ever memorable September 17. . . its day of strife and its night of death. Then followed the six weeks of rest to the army and unrest to the country, for in those days every man felt himself fully competent to comprehend the situation and dictate if he were not called to direct. And I, too, in my littleness and weakness, felt that something more remained for *me* to do and asked for 3 army wagons to proceed again to Harper's Ferry where Rumor predicted the forces would next engage.

My request was twice granted. They gave me *six* and an ambulance, and in the sun and dust of a dry hot October day in Washington I superintended the loading of them and at 2 o'clock ordered my little train to move out on the same road I had traveled a few weeks earlier to Antietam.

There may be those present who are curious to know how 8 or 10 stout, rough men, who knew nothing of me, received the fact that they were to drive their teams under charge of a lady. This question has been so often asked me privately that I deem it proper to answer it publicly. Well, a little oddly, not to say disdainfully. The various expressions of their faces afforded a study. They were not soldiers, but civilians in Government employ: *Drovers, butchers, hucksters, mule-breakers.* Probably not one of them had ever passed an hour in what could be termed *ladies society* in his life. But every man had driven thro' the whole Peninsular Campaign. Every one had taken his team unharmed out of that retreat and sworn an oath never to drive another step in Virginia. They were brave and skillful, understood their business to perfection but had no art. They said, and looked, what they thought, and I understood them at a glance.

They mounted and followed their leader, and I followed them. As early as 4 o'clock, they turned into a field, formed a circle, and prepared to camp.

I sent for the leader and inquired his purpose. With some surplus of English he assured me that "He wasn't going to drive in the night." I replied that he "could drive *till* night and he would find it for his interest to do so," and I said no more. By some course of reasoning he seemed to arrive at the same conclusion, for after a few minutes' consultation with the men, who stood grouped about their wagons cracking their long whips as a kind of safety valve to their smothered indignation, they drew their teams out into the road and moved on at a speed by no means retarded by their late adventure, and with the full measure of human perversity they not only drove till night but far into it.

But as they were moving in the right direction and working off their surplus energies I did not interfere with them. They evidently *wanted* to drive a little while after they had been ordered to stop. But I was not disposed to gratify them, and about 9 o'clock, getting weary of their fun, they halted beside a field and announced their intention of camping for the night. They had 8 days' dry rations of meat and bread in the feed boxes upon which they expected to subsist, cold and with little cooking.

While they were busy with their animals, with the aid of my ambulance driver a fire was kindled (these were the days when fence rails suffered) and I prepared a supper, which I now think would grace a well-spread table, but as I had no table, I spread my cloth upon the ground, poured the coffee, and sent my driver to call the men to supper. They came—a little slowly, and not all at once—i.e., they did not come upon me with a rush, but as I cordially assigned each one his place he took it, and I took my seat with them and ate and chatted as if nothing had happened. They were not talkative but respectful, ate well, and when through retreated in better order than they came.

I washed my dishes and was spending the last few moments by the broad bed of coals, for it was chilly, when I saw this whole body of men emerge from the darkness and come towards me. As they approached, I received them graciously and invited them to sit by the fire. They halted, reminding one of a band of Brigands with the red glare of the embers lighting up their brown, hard faces, and confronting me in silence awaited the spokesman. It was, of course, their leader George,[31] whose coal black hair and eyes would [have] well befitted the chief of a Banditti. As they waited, I again invited them to sit by the fire.

"No thank you," he replied, "we didn't come to warm us, we are used to the cold." "But," he went on slowly, as if it were a little hard to say, "But we come to tell you that we're ashamed of ourselves." I thought honest confession good for the soul and did not interrupt him. "The truth is," he continued, "In the first place we didn't want to come. There's fightin' ahead, and we've seen enough o' that for men who don't carry no muskets, only whips, and then we never seen a train under charge of a woman afore, and we couldn't understand it and we didn't like it and we thought we'd break it up, and we've been mean and contrary all day and said a good many hard things and you've treated us like gentlemen. We hadn't no right to expect that supper from you—a better meal than we've had in two years—and you've been as polite to us as if we'd been the Gineral and his staff. And it makes us ashamed, and we've come to ask your forgiveness. We shan't trouble you no more."

My forgiveness was easily obtained. I reminded them that as men it was their duty to go where there country had need of them. As for my being a woman, they would get accustomed to that, and [I] assured them that so long as I had food, I should share it with them. That when they were hungry and supperless *I* should be; that if *harm* befell them I should care for them; if *sick*, I should nurse them; and that under all circumstances, I should treat them like gentlemen. They listened silently, and when I saw the rough woolen coat sleeves drawing across their faces it was one the best moments of my life. Bidding me "good-night" they withdrew, excepting the leader, who went to my ambulance, hung a lighted lantern in the top, arranged the few quilts inside for my bed, assisted me up the steps, buckled the canvas down snugly outside, covered the fire safely for morning, wrapped his blanket about him, and laid down on the ground a few feet from me.

At daylight, I became conscious of the presence of low voices and stifled sounds and soon discovered that these men were endeavoring to speak low and feed and harness their teams quietly not to disturb me. On the other side I heard the crackling of blazing chestnut rails and rattling of dishes, and George came with a bucket of fresh water to undo my buckled door latches and announce that breakfast was nearly ready. *I had cooked my last meal for my drivers.* These men remained with me six months[32] thro' *frost*, and *snow*, and *march*, and *camp*, and *battle*, *nursed the sick*, *dressed the wounded*, soothed the *dying*, and buried the *dead*, and if possible grew kinder and gentler every day.

On reaching Harper's Ferry, Lee's army had slipped away, and Genl. McClellan had decided to follow them. Our Army was in the act of crossing the pontoon bridge at Berlin when we came up with it. We joined and crossed with them, and I found myself [at] once in the endless train of a moving army.

If time permitted, I should like to tell you of those grand old marches down beside the Virginia mountains following the lead of Pleasanton's Cavalry[33] skirmishing ahead, finding the enemy every day—those bright autumnal days—and at night the blaze of a thousand camp-fires lighting up the forest tops while from 10,000 voices rang out the never-ending chorus of the Union Army.

> John Brown's body lies mouldering in the grave
> While we go marching on.[34]

And thus on, day after day, no one knew whither till the rich autumn tints whitened in the frosts of an approaching winter and the merry brooks that laughed and leaped in the noon-day sun snuggled quietly into their beds at night under blankets of crystal. On and on (we were Burnside's Army now)[35] till finally we found ourselves beside a broad muddy river, and a little canvas city grew up in a night upon its banks. And here we sat and waited "while all the world wondered." Ay! it did more than wonder! It murmured, it grumbled, it cried shame shame to sit there and shiver under canvas. Cross over the river[36] and occupy those brick houses on the other shore. The murmurs grew to clamor and were fast deepening into disgrace.

Our gallant leader heard them and his gentle heart grew sore—he looked upon his army that he loved as it loved him—he looked upon those fearful heights beyond. Carelessness or incapacity at the capitol[37] had baffled his best laid plans till time had made his foes a wall of adamant, for

> Secure the Rebel's watchful care
>   had firm defences made,
> Breastwork and rampart work were there
>   and bristling palisade.
> Where nature well with craggy brow
>   her fences had begun
> The beetling cliff is frowning now,
>   with many a gaping gun.
> If ere security might lie
>   in steep assent of mountain high

In leveled gun and palisade, and marksman's
aim from ambuscade,
The Rebel troops in safety lay, on Frederick's
height that dreadful day.[38]

Still the country murmured—you friends have not forgotten how—for those were the dark days of old Fredericksburg and our little canvas city was Falmouth. Finally, one soft, hazy winter's [day] the army prepared for an attack. But here was neither boat nor bridge, and the sluggish tide rolled dark between. Hooker & Franklin were right and left, but here in the center come the brave men of the silvery haired Sumner.[39] Drawn up in line they wait in the beautiful grounds of the stately mansion whose owner, Lacy, had long sought the other side, and stood that day aiming engines of destruction at the home of his youth and the graves of his household.[40] There on the second portico I stood and watched the engineers as they moved forward to construct a pontoon bridge from the lower edge of the garden terrace to the sharp bluff on the opposite shore.

A few boats were fastened, and the men marched quickly on with timbers and plank. For a few rods it proved a success, and scarcely could the impatient troops be restrained from rending the air with their shouts of triumph. On march the little band with brace and plank but never to be laid by them. A rain of musket balls has swept their ranks, and the brave fellows lie level with the bridge or float down the stream.

No living thing stirs on the opposite bank—no enemy is in sight. Whence comes this rain of death? Maddened by the fate of their [comrades,] others seize the work and march onward to their doom, for now the balls are hurtling thick and fast—not only at the bridge but over and beyond to the limit of their range, crashing through the trees, the windows and doors of the Lacy House, and ever here and there a man drops in the waiting ranks silently as a snow flake, and his comrades bear him in for help or back for a grave.

There on the lower bank under a *slouched hat* stands the man of honest heart and genial face that a soldier could love and honor even thro' defeat, *the ever trusted, gallant Burnside.* Hark! that deep toned order rising above the heads of his men, "Bring the guns to bear and shell them out." Then rolled the thunder and the fire. For two long hours the shot and shell hurled thro' the roofs and leveled the spires of Fredericksburg.

Then the little band of engineers resumed its work, but ere ten paces of the bridge were gained they fall like grass before the scythe. For an instant all stand aghast. Then ran the murmurs, the cellars are filled with sharp-shooters and our shell will never reach them.

But once more over the heads of his men rose that deep-toned order, "*Man the boats.*" Into the boats like tigers sprang the 7th Mich[igan]. Row!! *Row*!! Ply for your lives boys, and they do. But mark them fall, some into the boats, some out. Other hands seize the oar and strain and tug with might and main. Oh! how slow the seconds drag, how *long* we *have held* our breath. Almost across, under the bluffs, and out of range. Thank God, they'll land. Ah yes, but not all. Mark the windows and doors of those houses above them. See the men swarming from them armed to the teeth and rush to the river. They've reached the bluffs above the boats. Down point the muskets. Ah! *that rain of shot and sheet of flame.*

Out of the boats, waist-deep in the water; straight thro' the fire—up, up the bank the boys in blue; grimly above, that line of gray. Down pours the shot, up up the Blue, till hand to hand like fighting demons they hang and wrestle on the edge. Can we breathe yet? No! still they struggle. Ah yes, they break, they fly up thro' the street and out of sight, pursuer and pursued.[41]

It were long to tell of that night crossing and the next terrible day of fire and blood. . . .[42]

But fearful as were the *great* events of those days, among their unwritten history are thousands of lighter incidents existing only in the memories of those who witnessed, as truly illustrative of the hour, as the 40 solid shot and mortar shell which poured the lurid light of day and the pale glimmer of the night thro' a single roof.

At 10 o'clock of the battle day when the Rebel fire was hottest, the shot rolling down every street and the ridge under heavy cannonade, a courier dashed over and rushing up the steps of the Lacy House placed in my hand a crumpled bloody slip of paper: a request from the lion-hearted old surgeon on the opposite shore establishing his hospitals in the very jaws of death. The uncouth penciling said, "Come to me. Your place is here."

The faces of the rough men working at my side, which 8 weeks before had flushed with indignation at the very *thought* of being controlled by a woman, grew ashy white as they guessed the nature of the summons, and the lips which had cursed and scowled in disgust trembled as they begged me to send *them* but *save myself.*

I could only permit them to go *with* me if they chose, and in 20 minutes we were rocking across the swaying bridge, the water hissing with shot on either side.

> Over into that city of death, its roofs riddled by shell,
> Its every church a crowded hospital,
> Every street a battle-line,
> Every hill a rampart,
> Every rock a fortress,
> And every stone wall a blazing line of forts.

Oh what a day's work was that! How those long lines of blue, rank upon rank, charge over the open acres up to the very mouths of those blazing guns and how like grain before the sickle they fall and melt away.

An officer stepped to my side to assist me over the debris at the end of the bridge. While our hands were raised in the act of stepping down, a piece of an exploding shell hissed thro' between us, just below our arms, carrying away a portion of both the skirts of his coat and my dress, ricocheting along the ground a few rods from us like a harmless pebble upon the water. The next instant a solid shot thundered over our heads, a noble steed bounded in air and with his gallant rider rolled in the dirt not 30 feet in the rear. Leaving the kind-hearted officer, I passed on alone to the hospital. In less than a half hour he was bro[ugh]t to me dead.

I mention these circumstances *not* as specimens of my own bravery. *Oh! no,* I beg you will not place *that* construction upon it, for I never professed anything beyond ordinary courage and a thousand times prefer safety to danger. But that those among you who have never seen a battle may the better realize the perils thro' which these brave men passed, who for four long years bore their country's bloody banner in the face of death and stood, a living wall of flesh and blood between the invading traitor and your peaceful homes.

In the afternoon of Sunday an officer came hurriedly to tell me that in a church across the way lay one of his men shot in the face the day before. His wounds were bleeding slowly and the blood drying and hardening about his nose and mouth. He was in immediate danger of suffocation. (Friends this may seem repulsive to you, but I assure you that many a brave and beautiful soldier has died of this alone.) Seizing a basin of water and sponge, I ran to the church to find the report only too true. Among hundreds of comrades lay my patient. For any human appearance above the shoulders it might as well have been anything else as a man—neither *sight*, nor *speech*, no *flesh* visible—all encased in one solid crust. I knelt by him and commenced with fear and trembling lest some unlucky movement close the last aperture for breath. After some half hour's labor, I began to recognize features. They seemed familiar. With what impatience I wrought. Finally my hand wiped away the last obstruction. An eye opened, and there to my gaze was the sexton of my own old home church. He is alive and well and scarcely carries a scar.

I have remarked that every house was a hospital. Passing from one to another during the tumult of Saturday, I waited for a regiment of infantry to sweep past on its way to the heights. Being alone and the only *woman* visible among that moving sea of men, I naturally attracted the attention of the old veteran Provost Marshal, Gen'l Patrick,[43] who, mistaking me for a resident of the city who had remained in her house until the crashing shot had driven her into the street, dashed thro' the waiting ranks to my side and bending down from his saddle said in his kindest tone, "You are alone and in great danger madam. Do you want protection?"

Amused at his gallant mistake, I humored it by thanking him as I turned to the ranks and adding that I believed myself to be the best protected woman in the United States. The soldiers nearest me caught my words and responding with "that's so, that's so," set up a cheer. This, in turn, was caught by the next line and so on, line after line, till the whole army joined in the shout, no one knowing what he was cheering at but never doubting there was victory somewhere. The gallant old general, taking in the situation, bowed low his bared head, saying, as he galloped away, "I believe you are right, madam."

It would be difficult for persons in ordinary life to realize the troubles arising from want of space merely for wounded men to occupy when gathered together for surgical treatment and care. You may suggest *that "all out of doors"* ought to be large [enough] and so it would seem, but the fact did not always prove so. Civilized men seek shelter in sickness, and of *this* there was ever a scarcity. 1200 men were crowded into the Lacy House, which contained but 12 rooms. They covered every foot of the floors and porticoes, lay on the stair landings. A man who could find opportunity to lie between the legs of a table thought himself rich; *he* was not likely to be stepped on. In a common cupboard with four shelves 5 men lay and were fed and attended. 3 lived to be removed and 2 died of their wounds. Think of trying to lie still and die quietly lest you fall out of a bed six feet high.

Among the wounded of the 7th Mich[igan] was one Wriley Faulkner, of Ashtabula County, Ohio, a mere lad, shot through the lungs and to all appearance dying when bro[ugh]t in. He could swallow nothing, breathed painfully, and it was with great difficulty that he gave me his name and residence. He could not lie down but sat leaning against the wall in the corner of the room. I observed him closely as I hurried past from one to another and finally thought he had ceased to breathe. At this moment another man with a similar wound was taken in upon a stretcher by his comrades, who sought in vain for a spot large enough to lay him down, and appealed to me. I could only tell them that when that poor boy in the corner was removed they could set him in his place. They went to remove him, but to the astonishment of all, he objected, opened his eyes, and persisted in retaining his corner, which he did for some (2) weeks, when finally, a mere little white bundle of skin and bones, for he gave small evidence of either flesh or blood, he was wrapped in a blanket and taken away in an ambulance to Aquia Creek to Washington with a bottle of milk punch in his blouse, the only nourishment he could take.

On my return to Washington, three months' later, a messenger came from Lincoln Hospital to say that the men of Ward 17 wanted to see me. I returned with him, and as I entered the ward 70 men saluted me, standing, such as could, others rising feebly in their beds and falling back, exhausted with the effort. Every man had left his blood in Fredericksburg. Every one was from the Lacy House. My hand had dressed every wound, many of them in the first terrible moments of agony. I had prepared their food in the snow and winds of December and fed them like children. How *dear* they had grown to me in their sufferings, and the 3 great cheers that greeted my entrance into that hospital ward were dearer than the applause that sounded sweeter than the voice of Josephine.[44]

I would not exchange their memory for the wildest hurrahs that ever greeted the ear of Conqueror or King. When the first greetings were over and the agitation had subsided somewhat, a young man walked up to me with no apparent wound, with bright complexion and in good flesh. There was certainly something familiar in his face, but I could not recall him until, extending his hand with a smile he said, "I am Wriley Faulkner of the 7th Mich[igan]. I didn't die and the milk punch lasted all the way to Washington!"

During the first day of the Battle of the Lacy House,[45] it will be remembered that the Rebel Army occupying the heights of Fredericksburg previous to the attack was very cautious about revealing the position of its guns. Consequently as the engagement became general on Saturday morning, their range must be obtained. The first shots were high, crossed the river, crashed thro' our house of wounded, and fell like hail among the reserves stationed about us. Of course, the reserves fell too and were bro[ugh]t in for medical care.

As I stood near the Eastern entrance a man apparently fainting was taken in by his comrades and lain upon the floor. A piece of shell had struck him near the ankle. At a glance I discovered that an artery was severed and he was rapidly sinking. The surgeons had nearly all been ordered over into the city, and of the few who remained not one was attainable. Making a tourniquet of my handkerchief, I succeeded in arresting the flow at the first trial, gave the poor fellow some stimulant, and left him to rest and wait for better skill. He chanced to lie near the passage leading from one room to another, and in the course of an hour as I passed by, I felt my dress held firmly by some obstruction. Terrified, lest it was caught on the helpless foot of some broken limb, I turned to find this poor, fainting man revived and holding on with all his strength to the skirt of my dress. He could not speak aloud, but the tears were sliding quietly down his brown, dust-covered cheeks. As I knelt to learn his wishes, he whispered faintly, "You saved my life." I smoothed back his tangled hair, wiped his face, and replied cheerfully that that was no matter. Did he want anything? "No."

An hour later as I passed the same thing occurred, and I was again informed in faint whispers that I had "saved his life." And so on, day after day, until he was removed. Whenever I came within reach of him I could feel my dress slipping gently thro' his fingers, and as often as he *dared*, he arrested me with the same four little words: "*You saved my life.*" Never seemed to want anything, and never said anything but this.

In all the confusion, I neither learned his name nor told him mine. He was taken away to hospital with others, and the circumstance nearly forgotten when one early spring day after my return to Washington, as I sat buried in the mass of accumulated correspondence, I heard a limping footstep in my hall and a rap at my door. I hastened to open it and there, leaning upon his crutch, stood my hero of the *four words*, and before I could recover from my surprise sufficiently to speak, he broke silence with "*You saved my life.*"

The soldier may well be reticent, for his is a life of *work, not words*. The world reads him in his glorious deeds, and the veteran of the Union Armies finds an example he may well follow, for the man of the fewest words in all America is the *soldier* who wears three stars.[46]

Friends, one evening is very little time and I must crave your pardon for the rapid journey of time I compel [you] to make while I pass from the old field of Fredericksburg in '62 to the later days of '64. The terrible slaughter of the Wilderness and Spotsylvania turned all pitying hearts and helping hands once more to Fredericksburg. And no person who reached it by way of Belle Plain, while this latter constituted the Base of Supplies for Gen'l Grant's Army, can have forgotten the peculiar geographical location and the consequent fearful condition of the country immediately about the landing, which consisted of a narrow ridge of high land on the left bank of the river. Along the *right* extended the river itself. On the *left*, the hills towered up almost to a mountain height.[47] The same ridge of high land [stood] in front at a quarter of a mile distant, thro' which at a narrow defile formed the road leading out and on to Fredericksburg, 10 miles away, thus leaving a level space, or Basin, of an area of a fourth of a mile, directly in front of the landing. Across this small plain all transportation to and from the army must necessarily pass.

The soil was red clay. The ten thousand wheels and hoofs had ground it to a powder and a sudden rain upon the surrounding hills had converted the entire basin into one vast mortar bed, smooth and glassy as a lake and much the color of light Brick dust.

The poor, mutilated, starving sufferers of the Wilderness[48] were pouring into Fredericksburg by thousands and all to be taken away in army wagons across this 10 miles of alternate *hills* and *hollows*, *stumps*, *roots*, and *mud*. The *boats* from Washington to Belle Plain [were] freighted *down* with *fresh troops* and back with supplies for the front. While the *wagons* from Fredericksburg to Belle Plain [were] loaded *down* with *wounded men* and back with supplies, and the exchange was transacted on this narrow ridge called the landing.[49]

I arrived from Washington about noon of the 8th [of May] with such supplies as I could take.[50] It was still raining. Some members of the

Christian Commission had reached [by] an earlier boat and being unable to obtain transportation to Fredericksburg had erected a tent or two on the ridge and were evidently considering what to do next. To nearly or quite all of them the experience and scenes were entirely new. Most of them were clergymen who had left at a day's notice by request of the distracted fathers and mothers who could not go to the relief of the dear ones stricken down by thousands and thus begged of him in whom they had most confidence and best loved to go for them. They went willingly, but it was no easy task they had undertaken. It were hard enough for old workers who commenced early and were inured to the life and its work.

I shall never forget the scene which met my eye as I stepped from the boat to the top of the ridge. Standing in this plain of mortar mud were at least 200 six-mule army wagons, crowded full of wounded men waiting to be taken upon the boats for Washington. They had driven from Fredericksburg that morning. Each driver had gotten his wagon as far as he could, for those in front of and about him had stopped. Of the depth of the mud the best judgment was formed from the fact that no entire hub of a wheel was in sight and you saw nothing of any animal below its knees and the mass of mud all settled into place perfectly smooth and glassy.

As I contemplated the scene, a young, intelligent, delicate gentleman, evidently a clergyman, approached me and said anxiously but almost timidly, "Madam, do you think those wagons are filled with wounded men?" I replied that they undoubtedly were and waiting to be placed on the boats then unlading.

"How long must they wait?" he asked. I said that "judging from the capacity of the boats, I thought they could not be ready to leave much before night."

"What can we do for them?" he asked still more anxiously.

I said, "they were hungry and must be fed."

For a moment his countenance brightened then fell again as quickly as he exclaimed: "*What a pity*! We have a great deal of clothing and reading matter, but no food in any quantity excepting crackers."

I replied that I had coffee and that between us I thought we could arrange to give them all hot coffee and crackers.

"But where shall we make our coffee?" he asked as he gazed wistfully about the bare wet hillside. I pointed to a little hollow beside a stump and said, "There was a good place for a fire and any of this loose brush will do."

"Just here?" he asked.

"Just here, sir."

He gathered the brush manfully and very soon we had some fire and a great deal of smoke, two crotched sticks, and a *crane*, if you please, and presently a dozen camp-kettles of steaming hot coffee. My helper's pale face grew almost as bright as the flames, and the smutty brands looked blacker than ever in his slim white fingers.

Suddenly a *new* difficulty met him. "Our crackers are in barrels, and we have neither basket nor box. How can we carry them?"

I said "aprons would be better than either," and getting something as near the size and shape of a common table-cloth as I could find, tied one about each of us, fastening all four of the corners to the waist and pinned the sides, thus leaving one hand for a kettle of coffee and one free to administer it. Thus equipped, we moved down the slope, and 20 steps bro[ugh]t us to the abrupt edge which joined the mud, much as the bank of a canal does the black line of water beside it. But here came the crowning obstacle of all. So completely had the man been engrossed in his work, so delighted as one difficulty after another vanished and success became more and more apparent, that he entirely lost sight of the distance and difficulties between himself and the objects to be served. If you could have seen the expression of consternation and dismay depicted in every feature of his fine face as he imploringly exclaimed, "How are we to get to them?"

"There is no way but to walk to them," I said.

One more look as much as to say, "And are *you* going to step in there?" I allowed no time for the question, but in spite of all the solemnity of the occasion and the terribleness of the scene before me, I found myself striving hard to keep the muscles of my face all straight, and the corners of my mouth would draw into wickedness as with a backward glance I saw the good man tighten his grasp upon his apron and take his first step in military life. But, thank God, it was not his last.

I believe it is recorded in *Heaven* the faithful work performed by that Christian Commission minister thro' long weary months of *rain* and dust and *summer's suns* and winter's snows. The sick soldier blessed and the dying prayed for him as thro' many a dreadful day he stood fearless and firm among fire and smoke not made of brush and walked calm and unquestioning through something redder and thicker than the mud of Belle Plain.

The early first soldier learned to view subjects from a standpoint so different from that of the civilian friend, who went *late* to serve him in his necessities that they were frequently at a loss how to comprehend each other. I recollect an incident of this nature which occurred at Point of Rocks when our army was pressing Petersburg in '64. The soldiers had lain in the trenches, soaked with water thro' one-half the season, till the burning suns of summer had dried the mud to the hardness of brick. And now they were scorching and baking and blistering thro' the other half.

An old veteran soldier, from a western regiment, had obtained leave to come down to the hospital and commission tents, in the hope of making some very *obviously* necessary additions to his wardrobe. I had been making the rounds of the hospital tents and for a moment stepped into the commission quarters, when this tall, sunburned, honest-faced soldier stepped in after me and approaching the agent said, "He should like to get a pair of stockings." The agent replied with great kindness that he was *very* sorry he could not oblige him, but they were out of stockings, excepting some very *fine* ones they had saved for *dead men.*

If you could have seen the look of puzzled astonishment which spread over that old veteran's face as he strove to comprehend the *meaning* of the reply. He looked at the agent, *at me*, at his own turtle-backed feet, innocent of stockings for months, until finally giving it up, he breaks out with, "*Stockings* for *dead men*," and turning on his heel, stalked out of the tent, no richer and apparently no wiser than he entered, doubtless back to the camp and trenches in disgust, and the young agent, who had been from home only a fortnight and had never learned by observation that men could lie quietly in their graves without stockings and shirts, was just as deeply puzzled to comprehend the astonishment of the soldier and stood gazing after him in silent wonder as he strode away. From their different standpoints, neither could get a glimpse of the other's thoughts any more than the good lady could understand how the war should increase the price of candles. "Candles higher!" she exclaimed, "Why bless me, do they fight by candle light?"

No person present has forgotten the heart sickness which spread over the entire country as the busy wires flashed the dire tidings of the terrible destitution and suffering of these same wounded of the Wilderness to whom I have alluded as they lay in Fredericksburg. But you may never have known how many hundred fold those ills were augmented by the unfortunate detail of improper, heartless, unfaithful officers to the immediate command of the city upon whose action and decisions depended entirely the *care, shelter, food, comfort* and *lives* of that whole city of wounded men. One of the highest officers I found there is since a convicted traitor. And another little dapper captain of 21, quartered with the owners of one of the finest mansions in the town, boasted that he had changed his opinion since entering the city in his present capacity the day before. "That it *was*, in fact, a pretty hard thing for refined people, like the citizens of Fredericksburg, to be compelled to open their houses and admit these dirty, lousy, common soldiers *and he was not going to compel it.*" This I heard him say and waited till I saw he made his words good and *did* not compel it, till I saw, crowded into one old sunken hotel,[51] lying helpless upon its *bare, wet, bloody* floors, *500* fainting men hold up their cold, dingy bloodless hands, as I passed, and beg me in Heaven's name for a cracker to keep them from starving, *and I had none*, or to give them a cup that they might have something to drink water from, if they could get it, and I had no cup and could get none. Till I saw 200 six-mule army wagons in a line ranged down the main street to head-quarters and reaching so far out on the wilderness road that I never found the end of it. Every wagon crowded with wounded men, stopped, standing in the rain and mud, wrenched back and forth by the restless, hungry animals all night, from 4 o'clock in the afternoon till 8 next morning, and how much longer I know not. But at that hour, as I passed for the last time down the fearful line, the dark spot in the mud under many a wagon told only too plainly where some poor fellow's life had dripped out in those hours of dreadful darkness.

A few of the faithful Sanitary [Commission] had reached [Fredericksburg], but they were powerless. A few volunteer surgeons had arrived, but they were also powerless, and the work grew upon their hands and the weight upon their hearts. Every door in the city, both stores and dwellings, barred like night, the haughty occupants holding barricade within and rejoicing at the suffering without. No order issued to open a house or take therefrom. The railroad and canal leading from the city, both closed, and only our half-vanquished and fighting army between the rebel forces and that city of helpless men. And no word had gone to Washington of all this.

I remember[ed] one man there who would set it right, if he knew it; who possessed the power and who would believe me if I told him. I demanded immediate conveyance back to Belle Plain, with difficulty I obtained it, and four stout horses with a light army wagon took me ten miles at an unbroken gallop thro' field and swamp and stumps and mud to Belle Plain, and a steam tug at once to Washington. Landing at dusk, I sent for Henry Wilson, Chairman of the Military Committee of the Senate. A messenger bro[ugh]t him at 8, saddened and appalled like every other patriot in that fearful hour by the weight of woe under which the nation staggered, groaned, and wept. He listened to the story of suffering and faithlessness and hurried from my presence with lips compressed and face like ashes. At ten he stood in the War Department. They[52] could not credit his report; he must have been deceived by some frightened civilian—no official report of unusual suffering had reached them. Nothing had been called for by the military authorities commanding Fredericksburg.

Mr. Wilson assured them that the officers in trust there were not to be relied upon. They were faithless, overcome by the blandishments of the wily inhabitants. Still the Department doubted. It was then he proved that my confidence in his firmness was not misplaced as, facing his doubters, he replied: "One of two things will be done: Either you will send some one to-night with authority to investigate and correct the abuses of our wounded men at Fredericksburg, or the Senate will send someone to-morrow."

This threat recalled their scattered senses. At 2 o'clock in the morning, the Qt. Master Gen'l[53] and Staff galloped to Sixth Street Wharf under orders. At *10* they were in Fredericksburg. At *noon*, the wounded were fed from the food of the city, and the houses were opened to the *dirty, lousy soldiers* of the Union Army. Both railroad and canal were opened. In three days, I returned with carloads of supplies.[54] No more jolting in army-wagons. And every man who left Fredericksburg by boat or car owes it to the firm decision of one man that his grating bones were not dragged 10 miles across the country or left to Bleach in the sands of that traitorous city. . . .

Notes

The following abbreviations appear in the notes.

AAS	Clara Barton Papers, American Antiquarian Society, Worcester, Massachusetts.
B	box
CB	Clara Barton
CBP	Clara Barton Papers, Library of Congress
F	folder
LC	Library of Congress, Washington, D.C.
OR	*War of the Rebellion: A Compilation of the Official Records of the Union and Confederate Armies.* 128 vols. Washington, D.C.: Government Printing Office, 1880–1901.
R	reel/roll

PREFACE

1. Miss H. P. Cleaves, "Clara Barton," February 22, 1913, speech delivered in Dorchester, Massachusetts, B156, R109, p. 60, CBP.
2. Hamilton, "Clara Barton," undated article at Andover-Harvard Theological Seminary, Harvard Divinity School, Cambridge, Massachusetts.
3. Brockett, *Lights and Shadows of the Great Rebellion*, pp. 341–342; E. R. Hanson, *Our Woman Workers*, p. 374.
4. Honora Connors to CB, February 15, 1897, B66, R54, pp. 60–63, CBP. The tradition that Clara Barton worked at Fredericksburg Presbyterian Church and at St. George's Episcopal Church likewise appear to be groundless. Alvey, *History of the Presbyterian Church*, pp. 42–43.
5. Dunn, "Clara Barton," pp. 244–245; Halsted interview, B70, R56, pp. 152–156, CBP; March 20–27, 1866, diary entries, R2, pp. 49–53, CBP.

CHAPTER 1. THE ANGEL OF THE BATTLEFIELD

1. Pryor, *Clara Barton*, p. 5; CB to Capt. J. W. Denney, B80, M63, pp. 26–30; CB, *The Story of My Childhood*, p. 21. Barton erroneously wrote that her father fought

under Wayne in the French and Indian War. See Barton, *The Story of My Childhood*, p. 20.
2. Pryor, *Clara Barton,* pp. 6–7, 40; CB, *The Story of My Childhood*, pp. 12, 23, 26, 99–100.
3. CB, *The Story of My Childhood,* pp. 12, 17–18.
4. Ibid., pp. 66, 72–74, 112–113.
5. Ibid., pp. 39, 49, 70–71, 77, 91.
6. Ibid., pp. 19–20.
7. Ibid., pp. 79–83.
8. Ibid., pp. 17–18, 27–32, 41–42, 94, 96–99.
9. Ibid., pp. 116–119.
10. Pryor, *Clara Barton*, pp. 22–23.
11. Ibid., pp. 23, 33–38, 48–50.
12. Ibid., p. 60; CB to Henry Wilson, September 29, 1865, B79, R63, pp. 17–18, CBP. Brockett and Vaughn, *Women's Work*, p. 113. For details on how Barton got this position and the harassment she endured there, see A.S.B., "How Clara Barton Kept a Secret," copy in B158, R110, p. 64, CBP. Barton's treatment at the hands of the new administration did not prevent her from attending Buchanan's levees. At one such party, she thought the outgoing president "looked happy," a fact she attributed to his "future release" from responsibility. CB to "My Dear Cousin," February 6, 1861, B2, F4, AAS.
13. CB to "My Dear Cousin," April 14, 1861, B2, F4, AAS. For additional evidence of Barton's pro-Unionist sentiments, see Brockett and Vaughn, *Women's Work*, p. 114; and CB to Thaddeus W. Meighan, June 24, 1863, B80, M63, pp. 43–48, CBP.
14. CB to B. W. Childs, 25 Apr. 1861, B2, F4, AAS.
15. Larcom, "Clara Barton, The Founder of the Society of the Red Cross," p. 252; CB to Peter H. Watson, undated letter, B80, M63, pp. 20–22, CBP. "I am a *U.S. soldier* you know," Barton wrote an acquaintance, "and therefore not supposed to be susceptible to *fear*,—and, *as I am* merely a *soldier* and *not* a *Statesman*, I shall make no attempt at discussing *political* points with you." CB to Thaddeus W. Meighan, June 24, 1863, B80, M63, pp. 43–48, CBP.
16. CB to B. W. Childs, April 25, 1861, B2, F4, AAS.
17. Pryor, *Clara Barton,* pp. 78, 81; "Letter from North Carolina," unidentified newspaper clipping, B157, R110, pp. 101–102, CBP; Brockett and Vaughn, *Women's Work*, pp. 115–116. According to Brockett, Barton's stock averaged five tons in early 1862.
18. Undated letter in B2, F4, AAS.
19. CB to J. M. Barton, July 21, 1861, B2, F4, AAS.
20. Oates, *A Woman of Valor*, p. 22; CB to "Sis Fannie," January 9, 1862, B2, F4, AAS; CB to Julia Barton, June 26, 1862, B2, F4, AAS.
21. Brockett, "Clara Harlowe Barton," p. 207. Barton had a twenty-four-inch waist. See CB to Annie Childs, November 1, 1863, B156, R109, pp. 39–41, CBP.
22. CB, speech draft in "War Lectures, 1860s" folder, B152, R107, p. 8, CBP.
23. Brockett and Vaughn, *Women's Work*, p. 117.
24. CB to John Andrew, March 20, 1862, B80, R63, pp. 11–12, CBP. The 21st

Massachusetts had departed Roanoke for New Bern, North Carolina, on March 11 but Barton may not have been aware of that when she submitted her request.
25. CB to Captain J. W. Denney, undated letter, B80, M63, pp. 26–30, CBP.
26. CB to Leander Poor, March 27, 1862, B2, F4, AAS; Note in "Memoranda" section of CB's 1862 diary, B1, R1, p. 74, CBP.
27. CB to Thaddeus W. Meighan, B80, R63, June 24, 1863, p. 46, CBP; CB to Leander Poor, May 2, 1862, B12, R9, pp. 6–9, CBP, original in B2, F4, AAS. Poor was a corporal in the United States Engineers.
28. CB to "Dear Bar," April 7, 1861, B2, F4, AAS. Barton was also on friendly terms with the Bay State's other senator, Charles Sumner, whom she considered "my advocate."
29. CB to Henry Wilson, January 18, 1863, B79, R63, pp. 3–4, CBP. Brockett and Vaughn, *Women's Work*, p. 118.
30. CB to "Dear Cousin," February 20, 1863, B2, F5, AAS.
31. CB to Henry Wilson, April 7, 1864, B1, R1, p. 55, CBP; CB to D. P. Holloway, December 11, 1863, B1, R1, pp. 16–18, CBP. In an odd twist of logic, Barton later insisted that *she* had done *him* a favor by allowing the man "to do my writing at one half the proceeds."
32. Brockett and Vaughn, *Women's Work*, p. 118.
33. CB diary, August 1, 1862; B1, R1, p. 46, CBP.
34. Pryor, *Clara Barton*, p. 89; Brockett and Vaughn, *Women's Work*, p. 647; "Massachusetts Women at Cedar Mountain," unidentified newspaper clipping in 1862–1864 Scrapbook, B157, R110, p. 94, CBP. Pryor spells her last name "Carner," while a correspondent with the *Boston Traveller* thought it was "Carney."
35 Shaver's obituary and other documents about him appear at the Find a Grave website: http://www.findagrave.com/cgi-bin/fg.cgi?page=gr&GRid=83740766.
36. "A Servant of God Called Home," undated article (ca. 1863–1864) published in the *American Baptist* newspaper; copy in B157, R110, pp. 98–99, CBP; *The American Annual Cyclopaedia and Register of Important Events*, 3:722; Brockett and Vaughn, *Women's Work*, p. 119. One writer called Welles "a young man of rare talent and devotion."
37. CB diary, August 2–3, 1862; B1, R1, p. 47, CBP.
38. Ibid. In a letter to his wife, Wolcott Marsh of the 8th Connecticut remembered Cornelius Welles occupying a tent near Chatham. Barton may have occupied a tent too or she may have stayed inside the house. Wolcott Marsh to "My Dear Wife," November 30, 1862, copy at Fredericksburg and Spotsylvania County Battlefields Memorial National Military Park.
39. CB diary, August 4, 1862; B1, R1, p. 47, CBP.
40. "Miss Clara H. Barton," unidentified newspaper article in B157, R110, p. 104, CBP; "Letter from North Carolina," undated *Worcester* (MA) *Spy* newspaper clipping, B157, R110, pp. 101–102, CBP. In a September 14, 1864, letter to her relative, Annie Childs, Barton called the 21st Massachusetts "the dear old regiment" and wrote that she "would divide the last half of my last loaf with any soldier in that regiment, tho I had never met him." Decades later, at the 21st Massachusetts's forty-fourth reunion, Barton told the aging veterans, "I do not merely wish to be

considered as a guest. This is my regiment." See "Letter Written by Clara Barton," *Worcester* (MA) *Sunday Telegram*, Sept. 16, 1917, and "Story of the Civil War," unidentified newspaper clipping in B157, R110, F478, CBP.

41. CB diary, August 5–11, 1862; B1, R1, pp. 47–48, CBP.

42. Ibid., p. 48; "Massachusetts Women at Cedar Mountain," unidentified newspaper clipping in B157, R110, p. 94, CBP. Relief agencies targeted their supplies and assistance to soldiers of specific states—in Tufts's case, Massachusetts.

43. "Massachusetts Women at Cedar Mountain," unidentified newspaper clipping in B157, R 110, p. 94, CBP.

44. Ibid.

45. Dunn mustered into service on March 6, 1862, as surgeon of the 109th Pennsylvania, but was later appointed surgeon of Brig. Gen. Henry Prince's brigade, which belonged to the Second Division of Maj. Gen. Nathaniel Banks's corps. See "Military Record of James Langstaff Dunn," Folder 13, in the James Dunn Papers, Special Collections, University of Virginia. Copies of Dunn's correspondence appear in Paul B. Kerr, *Civil War Surgeon: Biography of James Langstaff Dunn, MD* (Bloomington, Ind.: Authorhouse, 2005).

46. Dunn, "Clara Barton," p. 244; CB diary, August 13–14, 1862; B1, R1, pp. 48–49, CBP.

47. CB diary, August 13–14, 1862; CB, "Work and Incidents of Army Life," B152, R107, pp. 208–221, CBP; hereafter referred to as "Work and Incidents." The body of this speech appears in Part II of this book.

48. "A Letter from Miss Barton," 1862–1864 Scrapbook, B157, R110, p. 94, CBP.

49. CB to "Dear friends," September 4, 1862; B75, R61, "Sa-Sh" miscellaneous, pp. 85–89, CBP; CB diary, August 15, 1862; B1, R1, p. 49, CBP; Brockett and Vaughn, *Women's* Work, pp. 279–282. Barton identified her other associates as Mrs. Morrell, Mr. Haskell, and Dr. Henry J. Alvord, secretary of the Michigan Relief Association. Anna Carver was not in Washington at the time and did not accompany the group.

50. CB to "Brother and Sister," August 31, 1862, B2, F4, AAS.

51. CB to "Dear Brother & Sister," B9, R7, p. 13, CBP; CB to "Dear friends," September 4, 1862, B75, R61, pp. 85–89, CBP.

52. CB to "Dear Brother & Sister," B9, R7, p. 13, CBP; CB to "Dear friends," September 4, 1862, B75, R61, pp. 85–89, CBP.

53. CB, "Work and Incidents."

54. Ibid.

55. CB to "Dear friends," September 4, 1862, B75, R61, pp. 85–89, CBP.

56. Oates, *A Woman of Valor*, pp. 71, 75; CB, "Work and Incidents."

57. CB, "Work and Incidents"; Elwell memoir, B2, F6, AAS. The author was unable to locate this letter among Clara Barton's correspondence.

58. *Annual Report of the Adjutant-General of the State of New York,* Serial 33, p. 61. In her diary, Barton wrote that she visited Armory Hospital on August 30. She apparently entered the information under the wrong date. See August 30, 1862, diary entry, B1, R1, p. 51, CBP.

59. CB, "Work and Incidents."

60. Ibid.
61. CB to "Dear friends," September 4, 1862; B75, R61, "Sa-Sh" miscellaneous, pp. 85–89, CBP.
62. CB, "Work and Incidents."
63. Moore, *Anecdotes, Poetry, and Incidents of the War*, pp. 244–245; CB to "Dear friends," September 4, 1862; B75, R61, "Sa-Sh" miscellaneous, pp. 85–89, CBP.
64. CB to "Dear friends," September 4, 1862; B75, R61,"Sa-Sh" miscellaneous, pp. 85–89, CBP.
65. Ibid.
66. CB, "Work and Incidents."
67. Ibid.; CB to "Dear friends," September 4, 1862; B75, R61, "Sa-Sh" miscellaneous, pp. 85–89, CBP.

CHAPTER 2. ANTIETAM

1. CB, "Work and Incidents."
2. CB, "Work and Incidents"; Brockett and Vaughn, *Women's Work*, p. 119; CB, "Work on the Battle-Field," B157, R110, pp. 95–96, CBP. According to Barton, a sergeant from Boston with the name of Field was also a member of the party.
3. CB, "Work and Incidents."
4. Ibid.; CB, "Work on the Battle-Field," B157, R110, pp. 95–96, CBP.
5. CB, "Work and Incidents"; Welles, "Missionary Labors on the Battle-Field," B157, R110, pp. 96–97, CBP. Barton did not specify which gap she used, but Welles specifically states that they used "the mountain gap where Gen. Reno was killed," i.e., Fox's Gap.
6. CB, "Work on the Battle-Field," B157, R110, pp. 95–96, CBP.
7. CB, "Work and Incidents."
8. Ibid.
9. CB, "Work and Incidents."
10. Welles, "Missionary Labors on the Battle-Field," R110, pp. 96–97, CBP.
11. Ibid.; CB, "Work and Incidents"; CB, "Work on the Battle-Field," B157, R110, pp. 95–96, CBP.
12. Welles, "Missionary Labors on the Battle-Field," B157, R110, pp. 96–97, CBP.
13. Dunn, "Clara Barton," pp. 244–245.
14. CB, "Work and Incidents." Barton later wrote that four operating tables stood on the Poffenberger front porch. This is certainly an error as the porch, which still stands, is not wide enough to accommodate even a single table.
15. CB, "Work on the Battle-Field," B157, R110, pp. 95–96, CBP.
16. Welles, "Missionary Labors on the Battle-Field," B157, R110, pp. 96–97, CBP; CB, "Work and Incidents"; Brockett and Vaughn, *Women's Work*, p. 120. Welles recalled twelve soldiers helping out; Brockett placed the number at twenty-five, while Barton recalled having no fewer than thirty assistants.
17. CB, "Work on the Battle-Field," B157, R110, pp. 95–96, CBP.
18. CB, "Work and Incidents."
19. Ibid.
20. Welles, "Missionary Labors on the Battle-Field," B157, R110, pp. 96–97, CBP.
21. CB, "Work and Incidents."

22. Ibid. For an unembroidered account of this episode, see Brockett and Vaughn, *Women's Work*, p. 121.
23. Welles, "Missionary Labors on the Battle-Field," B157, R110, pp. 96–97, CBP.
24. Ibid.; Brockett and Vaughn, *Women's Work*, p. 121.
25. Welles, "Missionary Labors on the Battle-Field," B157, R110, pp. 96–97, CBP.
26. Ibid.
27. "Letter from the late Surgeon of the 124th Regiment, P.V.," unidentified newspaper clipping in B157, R110, p. 95, CBP.
28. Leander Poor to Elvira Stone, September 3, 1862, B2, F4, AAS. This letter seems to be misdated. It appears to have been written in October.

CHAPTER 3. FREDERICKSBURG

1. Nicolay and Hay, *Abraham Lincoln: A History*, 6:175. Lincoln's companion that day was Ozias M. Hatch, Secretary of State for the State of Illinois.
2. Memorandum at beginning of 1863 diary, B1, R1, p. 4, CBP; Brockett and Vaughn, *Women's Work*, p. 121. Barton later claimed to have supervised "8 or 10 stout, rough" men—meaning the teamsters. She may have had as many as seven teamsters—one for each vehicle—but it is unlikely she had more than that. If Stephen Barton and Cornie Welles each drove an ambulance, she would have needed only five, the number mentioned in her diary.
3. For Barton's highly embellished version of this event, see the Appendix.
4. Brockett and Vaughn, *Women's Work*, p. 121. At that time Harpers Ferry was still in Virginia. West Virginia would not formally become a state until June 20, 1863.
5. Memorandum in January–February 1863 diary, B1, R1, pp. 4–5, CBP.
6. CB to the Ladies of the Soldier's Relief Association of Watkins, New York, December 3, 1862 (*sic*: January 3, 1863), B156, R109, pp. 43–44, CBP; Samuel Barton to "My dear Cousin" (Elvira Stone), December 3, 1862, B14, R10, pp. 96–99, CBP; Brockett and Vaughn, *Women's Work*, p. 122; Walcott, *History of the Twenty-first Regiment, Massachusetts Volunteers*, p. 214.
7. Samuel Barton to "My dear Cousin" (Elvira Stone), December 3, 1862, B14, R10, pp. 96–99, CBP.
8. Ibid.; "Letters from Bro. Welles," undated newspaper clipping in B157, R110, pp. 97–98, CBP; Brockett, *Women's Work*, p. 122. Harriet Eaton, an agent of the Maine Camp Hospital Association, noted seeing "Mrs. Barton with her supplies" in Washington on December 2. Barton was still in the capital the following day when she wrote to her cousin Elvira Stone. See Schultz, *This Birth Place of Souls*, p. 86.
9. CB to Z. Brown, December 8, 1862, B80, R63, pp. 24–26, CBP.
10. Ibid.; "Letters from Bro. Welles," undated newspaper clipping in B157, R110, pp. 97–98, CBP. Barton later wrote that she departed for Fredericksburg the day after her arrival at Aquia Landing and infers that Welles accompanied her. Welles, by contrast, recalled spending two days at Aquia passing out supplies. The only way to reconcile the two statements is if Welles distributed his goods the day that he and Barton arrived at Aquia and again the following morning before they departed for Falmouth Station. Neither Barton nor Welles explicitly states how they got to Falmouth Station, although they almost certainly took the train.

11. CB to Z. Brown, December 8, 1862, B80, R63, pp. 24–26; Samuel Barton to "My dear Cousin" (Elvira Stone), December 3, 1862, B14, R10, pp. 96–99, CBP.
12. CB to Z. Brown, December 8, 1862, B80, R63, pp. 24–26. In the 1880s Sturgis sent Barton a basket of flowers with a note of praise to which she replied: "It is not that commendation is new to me, that this overcomes me. It is not that you speak me fair words of praise; I am used to that. It is not that you accord me a place in the grateful remembrance of our heroes, alive or dead; I am used to that. It comes from me from all sides and all sources, through all the years. But, General, it is that you, who knew me, who saw me, who helped me, who knew the helplessness of a woman alone in an army like that, who shielded me with kindness when a word, a look could have crushed me. It is that *you* should say it; that you should turn artist and paint my picture for your dead soldiers that rains the tears on my face, your 'Well done, good and faithful servant,' that melts me like a snowflake and humbles me like a child." See Hanson, *Our Woman Workers*, p. 374.
13. CB to Z. Brown, December 8, 1862, B80, R63, pp. 24–26. Sturgis's headquarters appears on a map of Union army camps in Stafford County found in the Warren Papers at the Library of Congress.
14. Ibid.; Schultz, *This Birth Place of Souls*, p. 92.
15. "Letters from Bro. Welles," undated newspaper clipping in B157, R110, pp. 97–98, CBP.
16. Clara Barton to the Ladies of the Soldiers' Relief Society of Watkins, New York; December [*sic*: January] 3, 1863, B156, R109, pp. 43–44, CBP.
17. "Letters from Bro. Welles," undated newspaper clipping in B157, R110, pp. 97–98, CBP. Welles added: "Cold, icy ground, with but a single blanket spread on it, makes an uncomfortable bed for a man racked with rheumatic pains, or rapidly declining with consumption stamped on every feature, or with typhus fever, burning pains, or debilitated and cold with long standing chronic dysentery. For all such cases we had something with which to comfort, even if we could not save life. When asked where these good things came from, we could tell them to thank Jesus, for it was he who inspired the hearts of the donors from the North, thus to remember the soldier, sick and disheartened on the field. While I was telling one young man from Stonington, Ct., who was in the first stage of recovery from typhus fever, that Christian hearts at home were thinking of him and praying for him, he burst into tears, exclaiming, 'Oh! I thought I was forgotten and forsaken, but Jesus remembers me still,' and then covering his face with his blanket, he wept like a child."
18. CB to Z. Brown, December 8, 1862, B80, R63, pp. 24–26, CBP.
19. CB to Elvira Stone, March 2, 1863, B14, R10, pp. 103–105, CBP.
20. CB to Elvira Stone, December 12 [*sic*: 11], 1862, B14, R10, pp. 99–101, CBP. The letter, written at 2 A.M., is dated December 12. However, the fact that she doesn't mention the bombardment and capture of the town suggests that it was actually written one day earlier. Barton's reference to "the roll of moving artillery" supports that theory. Union artillery moved into position to cover the pontoon crossing before dawn on December 11. It was largely in place by December 12. The "kind hearted general" referred to in the letter was not Ambrose Burnside, as has often been assumed, but rather Samuel Sturgis. For a typescript copy of the letter, see B156, R109, pp. 30–31, CBP.

21. CB to Elvira Stone, March 2, 1863, B14, R10, pp. 103–105, CBP; Pryor, *Clara Barton*, p. 105.
22. CB to the Ladies of the Soldiers' Relief Society of Watkins, New York; December [*sic*: January] 3, 1863, letter, B156, R109, pp. 43–44, CBP; untitled speech found in B152, R107, pp. 161–182, CBP; hereafter referred to as CB, "Fredericksburg." The heart of this speech has been reproduced in the appendix of this book.
23. CB, "Fredericksburg."
24. Note in 1863 diary, B1, R1, p. 26, CBP. Rosters for the 57th New York list no captain by the name of Perkins. The officer in question was almost certainly Capt. Augustus S. Perkins of the 50th New York Engineers, who died on December 11 while supervising the construction of a pontoon bridge below Chatham. See *OR* 21:170.
25. William Barton, *The Life of Clara Barton*, 1:300–301.
26. Barton told her friend Mary Norton that she was the only woman present at the Lacy House both during and after the battle. That is not true. Harriet Eaton was there and perhaps others. Lieutenant J. E. Hodgkins of the 19th Massachusetts wrote a letter from the house shortly after the battle telling the folks back home that he had "Received kind attention from the lady nurses who bring us some luxuries, sent by kind friends in the north." CB to Mary Norton, January 19, 1863, Norton Papers, Duke University; Turino, *The Civil War Diary of Lieut. J. E. Hodgkins*, p. 20; Schultz, *The Birth Place of Souls*, p. 92.
27. CB to Mrs. Carslake, March 29, 1863, B80, R63, pp. 37–38, CBP.
28. Ibid.
29. *OR* 21:614; Alexander, *Military Memoirs of a Confederate*, p. 296; CB, "Fredericksburg"; Schultz, *The Birth Place of Souls*, p. 92.
30. Murphey, "Reminiscences," pp. 30 ff.
31. Dyer, *The Journal of a Civil War Surgeon*, p. 53. Accounts of Confederate artillery shells striking the Lacy House do not agree. A correspondent for the *Philadelphia Sunday Dispatch* wrote that a shell struck the building just above the portico, where a band was playing "Bully for You." "This was the only shot that struck the building during the battle," he wrote, "and it did very little injury." Two other eyewitness accounts of this incident indicate that the shell burst over the regiment rather than striking the building. Both Josiah Murphey and Surgeon J. Franklin likewise remembered just one shell striking the house, but Murphey recalled the event occurring on December 13, while Dyer remembered it happening on December 15. In her speeches, Clara Barton inferred that several shells struck the building on December 13, while Surgeon John L. Brinton, by contrast, claimed that "although within range, this building under protection of the Hospital flags, was at all times respected." See "The Lacy House," *Philadelphia Sunday Dispatch*, January 18, 1863; Bliss, "Types and Traditions," pp. 520–521; Walcott, *History of the Twenty-first Massachusetts Volunteers*, p. 240; Brinton, "History of the Army of the Potomac," National Archives.
32. CB, "Fredericksburg."
33. Ibid.; Cornelius Welles to CB, undated note, B1, R1, p. 30, CBP; Lord, *History of the Ninth Regiment New Hampshire Volunteers*, p. 225. Barton's biographers

identify the surgeon as Calvin Cutter of the 21st Massachusetts. Cutter was in Fredericksburg that morning, but it is unthinkable that he would have summoned a woman to enter a city that was under fire. Barton surely knew better. She may have made the mistake unintentionally, but the fact that she avoided mentioning Welles and other aid workers in her speeches suggests that she changed the facts on purpose in order to focus attention on herself and to heighten the importance of the call. Barton claimed she received the note at 10 A.M., but this is too early as the Union attacks against Marye's Heights did not commence until almost two hours later. See "The Operations of Saturday," *New York Daily Tribune*, December 15, 1862, p. 1, and *OR* 21:574.

34. CB, "Fredericksburg."

35. Brockett, "Clara Harlowe Barton," p. 206; Brockett and Vaughn, *Women's Work*, p. 124.

36. Note in 1863 diary, B1, R1, p. 22, CBP.

37. CB, "Fredericksburg." For evidence that Confederate artillery shelled the town at this time, see *OR*, 21:576; Dyer, *The Journal of a Civil War Surgeon*, p. 53.

38. Linus Brockett's assertion that Barton "was the lady-superintendent of the hospital of the Ninth Army Corps" has no basis in fact. She had no official position in the army, either then or later. See Brockett, "Clara Harlowe Barton," p. 204.

39. Report of Dr. P. A. O'Connell, Ninth Corps Medical Director, in Record Group 94, Entry 544, Reg. No. 95, National Archives; John Bailey, December 13, 1862, diary entry, New Hampshire Historical Society, published in Lord, *History of the Ninth Regiment New Hampshire Volunteers*, p. 225. Although Cutter established temporary hospitals in town, the primary hospital for his division was near the Phillips house in Stafford County.

40. CB, "Fredericksburg"; Brockett, *Lights and Shadows*, p. 341; "Letters from Bro. Welles," undated newspaper clipping in B157, R110, pp. 97–98, CBP. Fredericksburg Baptist Church stands at the southeast corner of Princess Anne and Amelia Streets. Although the precise location of her kitchen will probably never be known, three candidates suggest themselves: the Wallace house, the Dr. Hall house, and the house of Mayor Montgomery Slaughter, each of which, like the Baptist Church, occupied a corner of the two streets. The Female Orphan Asylum stood two blocks west of the church, at the northeast corner of Charles and Amelia Streets.

41. "Letters from Bro. Welles," undated newspaper clipping in B157, R110, pp. 97–98.

42. CB, "Fredericksburg"; Untitled speech on Fredericksburg, on R107, F430, CBP.

43. Patrick, *Inside Lincoln's Army*, pp. 189–190.

44. For Barton's brief notation on her conversation with Page, see Barton's June 3, 1863, diary entry, B1, R1, CBP.

45. *OR* 21:327.

46. See Oates, *A Woman of Valor*, p. 113.

47. "Letters from Bro. Welles," undated newspaper clipping in B157, R110, pp. 97–98; Elwell memoir, B2, F6, AAS.

48. CB, "Fredericksburg." This incident appears in several places throughout Clara Barton's Papers. See B152, R107, p. 168, CBP. The "old home church" to which

Barton referred was the Old South Church of Worcester, Massachusetts. See undated note in Barton's 1862 diary, B1, R1, p. 13, CBP.
49. Barton identified Rice in an undated note scribbled in her diary. See B1, R1, p. 13, CBP.
50. *Massachusetts Soldiers, Sailors, and Marines in the Civil War*, 2:625; Walcott, *History of the Twenty-First Massachusetts Volunteers*, p. 251.
51. CB to the Ladies of the Soldier's Relief Association of Watkins, New York, December 3, 1862 (*sic*: January 3, 1863), B156, R109, pp. 43–44, CBP. The men of Sturgis's division were taken to Cutter's hospital, which was located at house of Alexander Phillips.
52. CB, "Fredericksburg."
53. Chatham had ten rooms at the time, one of which was used as the surgery. A basement stretched beneath the length of the building, but there is no evidence that soldiers were sheltered there.
54. CB, "Fredericksburg"; Dyer, *The Journal of a Civil War Surgeon*, p. 52. Barton informed a group of women in New York: "I cannot tell you the numbers but some hundreds of the worst wounded men I have ever seen, lying on a little hay on floors or in tents, and among these sufferers my dear ladies were used your gifts. I cannot tell you how gratefully they were received, or how much comfort they apparently contributed, but quite enough I am certain to satisfy generous and self sacrificing hearts like yours for any labor you may have performed, or sacrifice you may have made." CB to the Ladies of the Soldiers' Relief Association of Watkins, New York, December (*sic*: January) 3, 1862, B156, R109, pp. 43–44, CBP.
55. Dyer, *The Journal of a Civil War Surgeon*, pp. 53, 55; Account of an anonymous Union soldier in R2, F49–53, CBP; Brockett, *Lights and Shadows*, p. 342. Temperatures in the District of Columbia for the period of December 13–16, 1862, were extremely mild, ranging from 36 to 68.5 degrees. In Fredericksburg, where temperatures are typically three to five degrees warmer than in Washington, it must have been positively balmy. However, that changed abruptly on December 17 when cold weather moved into the area. Over the next five nights temperatures plummeted into the twenties and teens. See Krick, *Civil War Weather in Virginia*, p. 80.
56. Dyer, *The Journal of a Civil War Surgeon,* p. 53; Samuel Barton to "My dear Cousin" (Elvira Stone), December 3, 1862; B14, R10, pp. 96–99, CBP; Brockett, *Lights and Shadows*, p. 342; Brockett and Vaughn, *Women's Work*, p. 123. In a letter to her political patron, Senator Henry Wilson, Barton noted that Hammond had furnished her with the spirits "some months ago," long before the battle. She told Wilson that she had distributed the bottles "among the poor Sufferers who were shot in Saturday's fight and left lying up on the field, until brought across the river under flag of truce on Tuesday night." Ragged Confederates had stripped many of these men down to their underwear in order to clothe themselves. What "little clothing was left" on the Union soldiers, Barton noted, was "saturated in blood and frozen firmly to them." See CB to Henry Wilson, January 18, 1863, B79, R63, pp. 2–4, CBP.
57. Dyer, *The Journal of a Civil War Surgeon*, p. xxiv; CB, "Fredericksburg." Barton later wrote of the wounded soldiers at the Lacy House: "I had prepared their food, in the snow and winds of December and fed them like children."

58. Dyer, *The Journal of a Civil War Surgeon*, p. xxiv. Dyer may have been thinking of Barton when he wrote of relief workers: "These outsiders may have good intentions, but they don't know how to do anything. . . . [T]he work that all these men and women do about the hospitals does not pay for the time necessarily spent in taking care of them and waiting upon them. They want ambulances to take them to and from their stopping places, men to wait upon them with all manner of things, and will insist that they are doing an immense deal of good. I have got a division hospital—it is neat, clean, well managed and all have enough to eat and drink and I would not have a woman about it for anything."
59. "Letters from Bro. Welles," undated newspaper clipping in B157, R110, pp. 97–98, CBP.
60. Notes in January–February 1863 diary, B1, R1, p. 15ff., CBP. Among those whom Barton cared for was Cpl. Boughton Hill, a forty-year-old soldier in the 59th New York. Hill had been struck in the knee, and his wound was so severe that it would not bear amputation. During one of her many trips through the house, Barton loosened his bandage. Hill died on December 19. The three Confederates were Capt. Thomas W. Thurman and Pvt. William Simmons, both of the 13th Mississippi, and a third soldier whom Barton misidentified as Maj. T. A. Patterson of the 3rd Virginia Cavalry.
61. Wiatt, *History of the Nineteenth Massachusetts Volunteer Infantry, 1861–1865,* pp. 35, 152, 180–181, 183, 403.
62 Weymouth, *Memorial Sketch*, p. 118; A. B. Weymouth to CB, December 7, 1882, B78, R62, p. 41, CBP; Margaret Hamilton to CB, February 15, 1903, and CB to Margaret Hamilton, February 24, 1903, both in B70, R57, pp. 7–9, CBP.
63. CB, "Fredericksburg." Government records give Faulkner's first name as either "Riley" or "Wiley." The spelling given here is that used by Barton.
64. *OR* 21:327; CB to U.S. Senate Committee on Military Affairs, February 22, 1863, B80, R63, pp. 30–32, CBP; CB diary, Volume labeled "April 2–July 23, 1863," B1, R1, pp. 5–6, CBP; Excerpt from postwar speech, B152, R107, pp. 101–104 and 450–467, CBP; CB, April 1885 letter to "dear friend," B79, R63, pp. 49–51, CBP; *Massachusetts Soldiers, Sailors, and Marines in the Civil War,* 2:620; Barton, *The Life of Clara Barton*, 1:227–230.
65. Brockett and Vaughn, *Women's Work*, p. 123.
66. CB to U.S. Senate Committee on Military Affairs, February 22, 1863, B80, R63, pp. 30–32, CBP; Walcott, *History of the Twenty-first Regiment, Massachusetts Volunteers*, pp. 241, 258.
67. January 1, 1863, diary entry, B1, R1, p. 4, CBP.
68. CB to Annie Childs, May 28, 1863, B66, R54, pp. 4–6, CBP.
69. CB, "Fredericksburg." Napoleon is said to have remarked that "The first applauses of the French people, fell upon my ear sweet as the voice of Josephine," his wife. See Abbott, *History of Josephine*, p. 168. The author is indebted to Sylvia Frank Rodriguez for the source of this quote.

CHAPTER 4. MONTHS OF FRUSTRATION

1. Barton, *The Life of Clara Barton*, 1:227; *Fitchburg* (MA) *Sentinel*, May 20, 1864; Samuel Barton to "Cousin Mary," January 18, 1863, B2, F5, AAS. Doe may have

been the presiding officer of the Navy Yard Soldiers and Sailors Aid Society in Boston, but this is not certain.
2. CB to Mary Norton, January 19, 1863, Norton Papers, Duke University; Barton, *The Life of Clara Barton,* 1:227.
3. O'Reilly, *The Fredericksburg Campaign*, pp. 478–488.
4. CB to Mary Norton, January 19, 1863, Norton Papers, Duke University; CB diary, "Jan.–Feb. 1863" folder, B1, R1, p. 6, CBP. Barton had planned to return to the army around January 28, but her trip was delayed. CB to Henry Wilson, January 27, 1863, B79, R63, pp. 2–4, CBP.
5. CB, "Where Were You from 1861 to 1865, and *Why?*" a speech delivered on January 31, 1888; B153, R108, pp. 2–6, CBP; Speech fragment, R109, F502, CBP. See also R107, F88, CBP; Hanson, *Our Woman Workers*, p. 374.
6. For examples of letters written by Barton from Washington during this period, see B156, R109, pp. 31–35, and B80, M63, pp. 30–40, both CBP. See also "Work on the Battle-Field," B157, R110, pp. 95–96, CBP.
7. For a sampling of such letters, see B80, M63, pp. 32–40, 89–91, CBP.
8. CB to David Barton, February 20, 1863, B156, R109, p. 32, CBP; CB to Henry Wilson, April 7, 1864, B1, R1, F53, CBP. David Barton's commission, dated March 12, 1863, is in R109, F673, CBP. It was signed by President Lincoln on March 12, 1863.
9. April 7, 1863, diary entry, B1, R1, p. 7, CBP.
10. CB to Elvira Stone, B14, R10, pp. 107–109, CBP.
11. 1863 diary entries, *passim,* B1, R1, CBP. For a sample of Barton's leisurely lifestyle while at Hilton Head, see her May 14–24, 1863, diary entries, B1, R1, CBP.
12. CB to Elvira Stone, July 11, 1863, B14, R10, pp. 115–118, CBP.
13. CB to "My Dear Cousin," July 16, 1863, B2, F5, AAS.
14. CB to Mr. Ritchie, July 12, 1863, B2, F5, AAS.
15. CB to "My Dear Cousin," July 16, 1863, B2, F5, AAS.
16. June 18–23, 1863, diary entries, B1, R1, CBP; CB to Annie Childs, October 27, 1863, B156, R109, pp. 37–38, CBP.
17. CB to Elvira Stone, August 30, 1863, B14, R10, pp. 124–127, CBP.
18. CB to David Barton, August 2, 1863, B2, F4, AAS.
19. Ibid.
20. John J. Elwell memoir, B2, F6, AAS.
21. CB to David Barton, August 2, 1863, B2, F4, AAS.
22. "Clara Barton," an unidentified 1870 newspaper clipping in B157, R110, p. 68, CBP; Smith, *Record of Service of Connecticut Men*, p. 398.
23. Elwell memoir, B2, F6, AAS; Voris, *A Citizen-Soldier's Civil War*, pp. 10, 131–132, and 207.
24. CB to Lt. Ritchie, July 14, 1863, B80, M63, pp. 49–52, CBP.
25. CB to Henry Wilson, April 7, 1864, B1, R1, pp. 52–55, CBP. She later wrote of her weeks on Morris Island: "My food [was] the mouldiest, wormiest crackers I had ever seen an army insulted with, my drink, the tide water that leached through the loose sands of the little island fast becoming a crowded cemetery, my shade from a scorching August sun, the friendly clouds that scud between us, my light at night

the moon, a dying camp fire, and the long glowing trail of fire that followed the deadly track of the enemies shell that hissed and shrieked and burst above us."

26. Brockett and Vaughn, *Women's Work*, p. 126; Pryor, *Clara Barton*, pp. 117–123; Leander Poor to Elvira Stone, B14, R10, pp. 128–130, CBP.

27. CB to Elvira Stone, August 30, 1863, B14, R10, pp. 124–127, CBP; Leander Poor to Elvira Stone, August 27, 1863, B14, R10, pp. 122–124, CBP; CB to Annie Childs, October 27, 1863, B156, R109, pp. 37–38, CBP; December 5, 1863, diary entry, B1, R1, CBP.

28. Leander Poor to Elvira Stone, September 5, 1863, B14, R10, pp. 128–130, CBP.

29. Captain Samuel T. Lamb to Lt. Col. James Hall, September 7, 1863, B80, M63, pp. 54–55, CBP.

30. E. W. Smith to CB, September 15, 1863, B80, M63, p. 55, CBP.

31. December 5–8, 1863, diary entries, B1, R1, CBP. Barton later tried to justify her obstinacy by claiming that Dix's nurses refused her admittance to their hospitals. In reality, Barton simply could not abide taking orders from them. For evidence of her hostility toward Gillmore, see December 7, 15, 19, and 23, 1863, diary entries, B1, R1, CBP.

32. December 5, 1863, diary entry, B1, R1, CBP; Brockett and Vaughn, *Women's Work*, p. 126; Pryor, *Clara Barton*, pp. 117–123.

33. CB to Doctors Brown & Duer, March 13, 1864, B80, M63, pp. 68–74, CBP; CB to Annie Childs, November 10, 1863, B2, F5, AAS.

34. Brockett and Vaughn, *Women's Work*, p. 126; Pryor, *Clara Barton*, pp. 117–123; December 31, 1863, diary entry, B1, R1, CBP.

35. February 14 and March 31, 1864, diary entries, B1, R1, CBP.

36. March 17 and March 19, 1864, diary entries, B2, R1, CBP; CB to Henry Wilson, April 8, 1864, B1, R1, p. 56, CBP.

37. April 1, 1864, diary entry, B1, R1, CBP. Interestingly, Barton did not consult Poor before seeking the appointment. CB to Henry Wilson, April 7, 1864, B1, R1, pp. 52–55, CBP.

38. March 25, April 14, and April 19, 1864, diary entries, B2, R1, CBP. See also April 14, 1864, diary entry in B1, R1, p. 59, CBP. News from the Southern Department contributed to Barton's ill humor during this period. On February 20, 1864, one of her friends, Brig. Gen. Truman Seymour, had engaged Confederate troops in battle near the town of Olustee, Florida. Seymour was routed, losing nearly 40 percent of his force. A congressional committee investigating the disaster concluded that the general was at fault, but Barton would not accept its verdict. Although she had no firsthand knowledge of the situation, she firmly believed that Seymour had been made a scapegoat for the defeat and that his superior and her nemesis Quincy Gillmore was to blame. The more she thought about it, the more bitter she grew. Later, when Senator Wilson dropped by to pay his respects, Barton "poured out the vials of my indignation in no stinted measure. I told him the facts," she wrote, "and what I thought of a comm[i]tte[e] that was too imbecile to listen to the truth when it was presented to them—that they had made themselves a laughing stock for even the privates in the service by their stupendous inactivity and gullibility—that they were all a set of dupes, not to say knaves." Barton's tirade

caught Wilson off guard. "He looked amazed," she remembered, "and called for a written statement." He never got it. Perhaps realizing that she had spoken without being in possession of all the facts, Barton did not pursue the matter further. April 14, 1864, diary entry, B1, R1, CBP.

39. April 21 and 23, 1864, diary entries, B2, R1, CBP.

40. April 25–26 and April 30, 1864, diary entries, B2, R1, CBP.

41. May 2 [*sic*: 9], 1864, diary entry, B2, R1, CBP. Between May 9 and May 16, Barton wrote her diary entries under the wrong dates. In each case, her entries are one week off. Her May 9 entry appears under the date of May 2, her May 10 entry appears under the date of May 3, etc.

42. May 5–7, 1864, diary entries, B1, R1, CBP.

43. May 7, 1864, diary entry, B2, R1, CBP.

44. CB to Edwin M. Stanton, April 29, 1864, B80, R63, pp. 75–76, CBP.

45. Orsel C. Brown to sister, May 25, 1864, letter, Brown Papers, New York State Library. See also Edward K. Russell to "My dear sisters," May 15, 1864, letter, copy at Fredericksburg and Spotsylvania County National Military Park.

46. Adams, *Doctors in Blue*, p. 58.

47. *Rochester Evening Express*, June 14, 1864; May 30, 1864, B80, R63, pp. 80–84, CBP. Barton likewise never could have worked for Dorothea Dix, according to her biographer and relative William Barton. "She had too clear ideas of her own, and saw the possibilities of too large a work for her to be content with any sort of long-range supervision." W. E. Barton, *The Life of Clara Barton*, 1:296.

48. "A Missionary Fallen," unidentified newspaper clipping in B157, R110, p. 98, CBP; "A Servant of God Called Home," undated clipping from *The American Baptist* in B157, R110, pp. 98–99, CBP.

49. CB to Mr. J. Conroy, March 11, 1864, in R109, F686, CBP. Speaking of Welles, Barton told the editors of *The American Baptist*: "It is wonderful! The hold he had on the hearts about him." CB to Drs. Brown and Duer, March 13, 1864, B80, R63, pp. 68–72, CBP.

50. "A Missionary Fallen," unidentified newspaper clipping in B157, R110, p. 98, CBP.

CHAPTER 5. RETURN TO FREDERICKSBURG

1. May 3 [*sic*: 10], 1864, diary entry, B1, R1, CBP.

2. Schouler, *A History of Massachusetts in the Civil War*, 1:298–301.

3. May 4 [*sic*: 11], 1864, diary entry, B1, R1, CBP; Wheelock, *The Boys in White*, pp. 185–186; Reed, *Hospital Life*, pp. 12–13.

4. May 4 [*sic*: 11], 1864, diary entry, B2, R1, CBP; Wheelock, *The Boys in White*, p. 186.

5. Reed, *Hospital Life*, p. 13; Wheelock, *The Boys in White*, p. 187.

6. Reed, *Hospital Life*, pp. 13–16; Wheelock, *The Boys in White,* pp. 187–188.

7. Reed, *Hospital Life*, p. 13.

8. CB, "Fredericksburg"; Untitled speech, R107, F432, CBP.

9. *OR* 36(2):737–738.

10. May 5 [*sic*: 12], 1864, diary entry, B2, R1, F534–41, CBP; Wheelock, *The Boys in White,* pp. 188–189.

11. A partial list of people who slept aboard the *Young America* on the night of May 12 appears in a memorandum at the end of Barton's 1864 diary, B2, R1, p. 104, CBP.
12. May 5 [*sic*: 12], 1864, diary entry, B2, R1, CBP; Wheelock, *The Boys in White*, pp. 187–188.
13. CB, undated speech, B152, R107, p. 433, CBP.
14. Ibid., p. 159.
15. Wheelock, *The Boys in White*, p. 189; Reed, *Hospital Life*, pp. 13–16.
16. May 6 [*sic*: 13], 1864, diary entry, B2, R1, CBP. Cruikshanks had been born in Haddington, Scotland, in 1828 and came to the United States at the age of fourteen. He graduated from Yale in 1855 and after studying for three years at theological seminaries he received his ordination at Everett, Massachusetts, in 1858. He became minister of Spencer Congregationalist Church just a few months prior to his appearance at Belle Plain. He died in Chicago in 1889. See Tower, *Historical Sketches*, 2:194–195; Moss, *Annals*, p. 638; Howard, *Religion*, p. 147; Carpenter, *Six Months at the White House*, p. 162.
17. CB, "Fredericksburg." In her diary Barton described the mud at the landing as "ankle deep." Yet in her later speeches, she asserted "that no *entire* hub of a [wagon] wheel was in sight, and you saw nothing of any animal below its knees." The latter statement seems to be the more accurate of the two. William Reed, too, wrote that the mud was "up to the wheel hubs," while Julia Wheelock recalled "wading through mud to the top of our boots." See Reed, *Hospital Life*, pp. 13–14, and Wheelock, *The Boys in White*, p. 189.
18. May 6 [*sic*: 13], 1864, diary entry, B2, R1, CBP. Keenan had been shot in the Wilderness on May 6.
19. Ibid.
20. May 7 [*sic*: 14], 1864, diary entry, B2, R1, CBP; *OR* 36(2):737. Barton placed the number of prisoners at 9,000, while Reed wrote that there were precisely 9,453. See Reed, *Hospital Life*, p. 17.
21. May 7 [*sic*: 14], 1864, diary entry, B2, R1, CBP; Reed, *Hospital Life*, pp. 16–19.
22. Reed, *Hospital Life*, p. 19; *OR* 36(1):236; Edward K. Russell to "My dear Sisters," May 15, 1864, copy at Fredericksburg and Spotsylvania County Battlefields Memorial National Military Park. Surgeons used red flags to denote buildings being used as hospitals.
23. Robert Corson to Hon. J. A. Gilmore, May 24, 1864, Executive Papers, New Hampshire State Archives, Concord, New Hampshire. On the need of straw for bedding, see *OR* 36(2):855 and Smith, *Incidents Among Shot and Shell*, p. 249.
24. Wheelock, *The Boys in White*, pp. 191–192.
25. CB diary, B1, R1, December 1862 folder, p. 3, CBP.
26. Adams, *Doctors in Blue*, p. 58; CB, undated speech, B152, R107, p. 197, CBP.
27. OR 36(1):235. Medical Director Thomas McParlin wrote that "The obstacles to the removal of the more seriously wounded by way of Belle Plain were very great, and it would certainly have caused the death of a large number had the removal been attempted. The road between that point and Fredericksburg was to a

considerable extent corduroy and very rough, nor could it be improved by any means then available."

28. CB diary, B1, R1, December 1862 folder, pp. 2–3, CBP. Tangs are the wooden beams that connect the ambulance's frame with the animals pulling it.

29. CB diary, B1, R1, December 1862 folder, p. 3, CBP. Dr. Alfred Hitchcock (1813–1872) of Fitchburg, Massachusetts, was a graduate of Dartmouth Medical School and a delegate of the Massachusetts state relief agency. He was present at Fredericksburg in May 1864 as a representative of the Citizen Committee of Fitchburg. He served on the Executive Council of Massachusetts from 1861 to 1863 and sat on the Board of Overseers for Harvard University from 1857 to 1865. See Emerson, *Fitchburg, Massachusetts, Past and Present*, pp. 81–82; Hurd, *History of Worcester County*, 1:303.

30. CB diary, B1, R1, December 1862 folder, p. 2, CBP; May 7 [*sic*: 14], 1864, diary entry, B2, R1, CBP.

31. Epler, *The Life of Clara Barton*, pp. 91–92. George Barton did not receive his captain's commission until July 20, 1864. *Massachusetts Soldiers, Sailors, and Marines in the Civil War*, 4:811.

32. December 24, 1864, diary entry, B2, R1, CBP. Barton called the building the "Old National Hotel." Her observation that the building contained "western men" identifies it as the hospital of Willcox's Third Division, which had an unusually large number of Michigan troops. Julia Wheelock, one of the Michigan Soldiers' Relief Association workers who journeyed with Barton to Belle Plain aboard the *Winona,* identified the hospital by its correct name, Planter's Hotel. See Wheelock, *The Boys in Blue*, p. 194.

33. Anecdote found in B152, R107, "Lectures and lecture notes, 1865–1868," pp. 84–85, CBP. Euchre is a card game. To be "euchred" is to lose.

34. CB diary, B1, R1, December 1862 folder, pp. 2–3, CBP; December 24, 1864, diary entry, B2, R1, CBP.

35. CB diary, B1, R1, December 1862 folder, pp. 2–3, CBP; "Letter from Frances D. Gage," *National Anti-Slavery Standard*, ca. June 1864; copy in R110, F363, CBP. For a more dramatic account of this episode, see CB, "Fredericksburg."

36. May 8 [*sic*: 15], 1864, diary entry, B2, R1, p. 41, CBP. It is not certain that Barton spent the night at the Christian Commission office, but a note in her diary, "to Christian C.," suggests that she may have done so. The Christian Commission had its Fredericksburg office in a large, deserted house owned by a man named Hart. National Park Service historian John J. Hennessy believes the building to be the William T. Hart house, which stood on Hanover Street, opposite the terminus of Charles Street. Unfortunately, the house no longer stands. *Huntingdon* (PA) *Globe*, June 29, 1864; *The United States Christian Commission for the Army and Navy*, p. 72.

37. CB diary, B1, R1, December 1862 folder, pp. 2–3, CBP; CB, "Fredericksburg." Compare Harrison, *Fredericksburg Civil War Sites*, 2:209–210.

38. CB, "Fredericksburg."

39. Ibid.

40. Ibid.

41. Ibid.
42. Ibid.; May 8 [*sic*: 15], 1864, diary entry, B2, R1, CBP; *Lowell* (MA) *Daily Citizen and News*, May 10, 1864. Hurd, *History of Worcester County, Massachusetts*, 1:242, 329. For Jones's rank and position, see *OR* 36(2):799. Goodrich had arrived at Fredericksburg on May 13 in the company of Dr. Alfred Hitchcock and Mr. E. B. Hayward. They departed the town on May 21. The three men constituted the Citizens Committee of Fitchburg, Massachusetts.
43. CB, "Fredericksburg."
44. May 8 [*sic*: 15], 1864, diary entry, B2, R1, CBP. For Pitkin's rank and position, see *OR* 36(2):799.
45. May 7–8 [*sic*: 14–15], 1864, diary entry, B2, R1, CBP; CB, "Fredericksburg."
46. CB, "Fredericksburg."
47. Stanton's dispatch to Meigs, written on May 16, 1864, at 11:40 A.M., ordered him to go to Fredericksburg and take command there. "You will, while at Belle Plain and at Fredericksburg, consider yourself the ranking officer in command and issue such orders as the police and safety of either place may require. You will go to Fredericksburg and inspect the different branches of the service there." *OR* 36(2):829. Meigs did not receive the message until 4:30 A.M. May 17. That evening he replied: "I have given orders for such arrangements for comfort and quick transportation of wounded and for their supply as seemed advisable and practicable. I wrote to General Grant in regard to the situation of the place." *OR* 36(2):854–855.
48. CB, "Fredericksburg." Barton was still in Washington at the time. How she knew these things she did not say.
49. *OR* 36(1):270.
50. "Interesting Army Correspondence," *Crawford Journal*, May 24, 1864; Burton, "Spotsylvania: Letters from the Field," pp. 22–26. Dawes, *Service with the Sixth Wisconsin Volunteers*, p. 256. George K. Chandler, a soldier in the Ninth New Hampshire, wrote his mother on May 17 from the home of Fredericksburg's mayor, Montgomery Slaughter: "I am having good medical attendance, and a[s] good care and nursing, as can be afforded under the present circumstances." George K. Chandler to "My Dear Mother," May 17, 1864, George Chandler Papers, New Hampshire Historical Society. Even Clara Barton's own cousin, Ned Barton, had been taken to a private home on May 11. Edward M. Barton diary, May 11, 1864, American Antiquarian Society, Worcester, Massachusetts.
51. *OR* 36(2):738, 770, 809–10, 812, 840.
52. *OR* 36(2):854–55. According to Barton, Wilson visited her on May 29, 1864, and told her that her trip to Washington had prompted the opening of the railroad. Wilson may have believed this, but evidence suggests that the army would have repaired the railroad anyway. May 29, 1864, diary entry, B2, R1, CBP.
53. Willis, *Fitchburg in the War of the Rebellion*, pp. 140–142; "From the Battle Fields," *Fitchburg* (Massachusetts) *Sentinel*, May 27, 1864. In a letter to Governor John A. Andrew of Massachusetts written from Washington on May 22, Hitchcock affirmed that "The deficiency of hospital and sanitary supplies no longer exists. The facilities and means of treating the wounded have been greatly improved within a few days. They are generally doing well." *Worcester National Aegis*, May 28, 1864.

54. May 9 [*sic*: 16], 1864, diary entry, B2, R1, CBP.
55. "Washington Correspondence," *Fitchburg* (MA) *Sentinel*, May 20, 1864.
56. May 9 [*sic*: 16], 1864, diary entry, B2, R1, CBP.
57. May 10 [*sic*: 17], 1864, diary entry, B2, R1, CBP.
58. May 11 [*sic*: 18], 1864, diary entry, B2, R1, CBP. Ferguson worked as a clerk at the Treasury Department. See *Register of Officers and Agents*, p. 17.
59. "A Call for the Suffering Wounded," *American Baptist* (New York), May 24, 1864, copy in B157, R110, p. 107, CBP.
60. May 11 [*sic*: 18], 1864, diary entry, B2, R1, CBP.
61. "Letter from Frances D. Gage," undated article in *National Anti-Slavery Standard*, B157, R110, p. 106, CBP.
62. CB to Mrs. Alling, May 30, 1864, B80, M63, pp. 80–84, CBP.
63. May 12–13 [*sic*: 19–20], 1864, diary entries, B2, R1, CBP.
64. May 11 [18], 1864, diary entry, B2, R1, CBP. Among the groups that sent Barton supplies through Tufts was the Citizens Committee of Fitchburg, Massachusetts. Its representatives informed the committee that they had forwarded the committee's supplies to Barton "to be distributed as she saw fit," adding that "her discretion wisdom and fidelity are well known in this State, as well as through the army of the Potomac." It is unlikely that Barton received the supplies before she left Fredericksburg, however. Willis, *Fitchburg in the War of the Rebellion*, pp. 140–142; "From the Battle Fields," *Fitchburg* (MA) *Sentinel*, May 27, 1864.
65. May 11–13 [18–20], 1864, diary entries, B2, R1, CBP.
66. January 1–4, 1864, diary entries, B2, R1, CBP. The comments under these dates are actually a continuation of Barton's May 1864 entries, starting on May 21.
67. January 1–4, 1864, diary entries, B2, R1, CBP; *OR* 36(1):152.
68. January 1–4, 1864, diary entries, B2, R1, CBP. The names of the Michigan delegates were Mr. Wallace and Mr. Wilcox. Barton noted that a Michigan colonel named Barnes was also in the party. She may have been referring to Maj. George C. Barnes of the 20th Michigan.
69. *OR* 36(2):770–771. Stanton undoubtedly feared that Northerners in search of wounded or dead relatives would flood the town.
70. January 1–4, 1864, diary entries, B2, R1, CBP.
71. Ibid.
72. Ibid. From 1862 to 1865 Lamb had worked at military hospitals in Alexandria, Virginia. After the war, while serving on the faculty of Howard University Medical School, he performed autopsies on President James A. Garfield and Garfield's assassin, Charles J. Guiteau. See https://www.flickr.com/photos/medicalmuseum/3300121774/. On the date of Hitchcock's departure, see Willis, *Fitchburg in the War of the Rebellion*, pp. 140–142.
73. Edward Barton, May 22, 1864, diary entry, Edward M. Barton Papers, American Antiquarian Society, Worcester, Massachusetts; January 1–4, 1864, diary entries, B2, R1, CBP.
74. Heitman, *Historical Register*, 1:866.
75. *OR* 36(2):770; Edward Barton, May 22, 1864, diary entry, Edward M. Barton Papers, American Antiquarian Society, Worcester, Massachusetts; January 1–4,

1864, diary entries, B2, R1, CBP.
76. January 1–4, 1864, diary entries, B2, R1, CBP. George Barton was actually Clara's first cousin once removed, being the grandson of her Uncle Giden. See CB to David Barton, May 26, 1864, B2, F6, AAS.
77. January 1–4, 1864, diary entries, B2, R1, CBP. For a biographical sketch of Isabella Fogg, see F. Moore, *Women of the War*, pp. 113–26.
78. January 1–4, 1864, diary entries, B2, R1, CBP; *OR* 36(1):271.
79. January 1–4, 1864, diary entries, B2, R1, CBP.
80. CB to Mrs. Alling, May 30, 1864, B80, R63, pp. 80–84, CBP.
81. CB to David Barton, May 26, 1864, B2, F6, AAS.
82. Ibid.

CHAPTER 6. THE ARMY OF THE JAMES

1. CB to Mr. Baldwin, May 30, 1864, B80, R63, pp. 79–80, CBP. Casualties in the Overland Campaign were indeed staggering, some regiments losing more than two-thirds of their number. However Barton's assertion that regiments that typically entered the campaign with three hundred or more soldiers were reduced to twenty and consequently were led by corporals is an exaggeration.
2. CB to David Barton, May 26, 1864, American Antiquarian Society, Worcester, Massachusetts.
3. Oates, *A Woman of Valor*, p. 244; Pryor, *Clara Barton*, pp. 126–127; June 21, 1864, diary entry, B2, R1, CBP. During her three years in the field, Barton served with the Department of the Rappahannock at Fredericksburg, the Army of Virginia at Culpeper Court House, the Army of the Potomac at Antietam and Fredericksburg, the Department of the South in South Carolina, and the Army of the James at Bermuda Hundred.
4. Bainbridge, "Three Pictures of Abraham Lincoln," p. 244; June 22, 1864, diary entry (listed under June 8), B2, R1, CBP.
5. Ibid.; June 23, 1864, diary entry (listed under June 9), B2, R1, CBP.
6. William Barton, *The Life of Clara Barton*, 1:293.
7. June 23, 1864, diary entry (listed under June 9), B2, R1, CBP; Pryor, *Clara Barton*, pp. 118–119; Smith, *Reminiscences*, p. 80. Barton described Butler as "dignified, wise, and princely, and still, perhaps the most kindly and approachable personage on the grounds." See "A Graphic and Excellent Letter from Clara Barton," undated newspaper clipping from the *New York Evening Express* found in B157, R110, p. 109, CBP.
8. William Barton, *The Life of Clara Barton*, 1:293. MASH is an acronym for Mobile Army Surgical Hospital.
9. June 23, 1864, and July 3, 1864 diary entries, B2, R1, CBP; "Surviving Veterans of 21st Mass. Regiment at 51st Annual Reunion," unidentified newspaper article in B157, R110, p. 13, CBP; CB to "My most esteemed & dear friend," July 5, 1864, B80, M63, pp. 84–87, CBP; Pryor, *Clara Barton*, 127; Brockett and Vaughn, *Women's Work*, p. 116. Of Barton, Brockett wrote: "She neither sought or received recognition by any department of the Government, by which I mean only that she had no acknowledged position, rank, rights or duties, was not employed, paid, or compensated in any way, had authority over no one, and was subject to no one's

orders. She was simply an American lady, mistress of herself and of no one else; free to stay at home, if she had a home, and equally free to go where she pleased."

10. CB to "My most esteemed & dear friend," July 5, 1864, B80, M63, pp. 84–87, CBP.

11. "A Graphic and Excellent Letter from Clara Barton," undated newspaper clipping from the *New York Evening Express* found in B157, R110, p. 109, CBP; Pryor, *Clara Barton*, p. 127; July 2, 5, and 6, 1864, diary entries, B2, R1, CBP; Smith, *Reminiscences*, p. 84; "Letter from Miss Clara Barton," undated newspaper clipping from the *Worcester Daily Spy* found in B157, R110, p. 110, CBP; CB to Elvira Stone, October 20, 1864, B14, R10, pp. 147–151, CBP; William Barton, *The Life of Clara Barton*, 1:291.

12. CB to "My most esteemed & dear friend," July 5, 1864, B80, M63, pp 84–87, CBP.

13. July 6, 1864, and August 4, 1864, diary entries, B2, R1, CBP; Pryor, *Clara Barton*, p. 128. For the quality of Barton's cooking, see Voris, *A Citizen-Soldier's Civil War*, p. 236.

14. September 30, 1864, and October 1, 1864, diary entries, B2, R1, CBP.

15. "Letter from Miss Clara Barton," undated newspaper clipping published in the *Worcester Daily Spy*, B157, R110, p. 110, CBP.

16. "A Graphic and Excellent Letter from Clara Barton," undated newspaper clipping from the *New York Evening Express* found in B157, R110, p. 109, CBP; October 1, 1864, diary entry, B2, R1, CBP.

17. "A Graphic and Excellent Letter from Clara Barton," undated newspaper clipping from the *New York Evening Express* found in B157, R110, p. 109, CBP. For additional evidence of the heat, see July 1, 2, and 31, 1864, and August 8, 1864, diary entries, B2, R1, CBP, and CB to "My most esteemed & dear friend," July 5, 1864, B80, M63, pp. 84–87, CBP.

18. July 3–5, 1864, diary entries, B2, R1, CBP. In September, Barton wrote: "I have not even a cook or orderly, not to say a clerk. I do not mean that I cannot have the two former, but I do not use them myself at all when I hold them in detail. I immediately get them at work for some one I think needs them more." William Barton, *The Life of Clara Barton*, 1:295.

19. Smith, *Reminiscences*, p. 78; Brockett, *Women's Work*, pp. 441–448; July 30, 1864, diary entry, B2, R1, CBP.

20. Smith, *Reminiscences*, p. 90; July 30, 1864, and August 3, 1864, diary entries, B2, R1, CBP. Barton departed Point of Rocks for Washington on July 15 and started back on July 28. See July 15 and 28, 1864, diary entries, B2, R1, CBP.

21. August 6–7, 1864, diary entries B2, R1, CBP.

22. Smith, *Reminiscences*, pp. 90, 93; August 5 and 8, 1864, diary entry, B2, R1, CBP. Under the dates of August 4–5, Barton wrote in her diary: "At night we picked up a lot of fish and had it for breakfast on Friday 5th. But the fatigue men were discontented at not having enough, and I felt hurt and retired for the day to try to decide if I were right to try to do anything or not—so I did nothing." See August 4–5, 1864, diary entries, B2, R1, CBP.

23. Pryor, *Clara Barton*, pp. 128–129.

24. CB to Elvira Stone, undated letter fragment (ca. late 1863) in B14, R10, pp. 139–141, CBP.
25. Voris, *A Citizen-Soldier's Civil War*, pp. 214–215.
26. Ibid., pp. 207, 209, and 213.
27. April 7, 1863, diary entry, B1, R1, CBP.
28. July 30, 1864, and August 1, 1864, diary entries, B2, R1, CBP; Oates, *A Woman of Valor*, p. 262; William Barton, *The Life of Clara Barton*, 1:292. Gardner and Clark served in the 21st Massachusetts, while Gould commanded the 59th Massachusetts. Gould would die of his wounds. For comments by Barton on Gardner, see "Story of the Civil War," unidentified newspaper clipping in "Scrapbooks, 1865–1929" file, B157, R110, p. 104, CBP.
29. "Story of the Civil War," unidentified newspaper clipping in "Scrapbooks, 1865–1929" file, B157, R110, p. 104, CBP.
30. August 8, 1864, diary entry, B2, R1, CBP.
31. Brager, "The City Point Explosion."
32. CB to "Sis Fannie," September 3, 1864, B2, F6, AAS.
33. Ibid.
34. September 28–29, 1864, diary entries, B2, R1, CBP.
35. September 28 to October 3, 1864, and October 12, 1864, diary entries, B2, R1, CBP.
36. CB to Elvira Stone, October 20, 1864, B14, R10, pp. 147–151, CBP; CB to "Ladies of the Soldiers Aid Society, West Fitchburg, Mass.," January 26, 1865, B80, M63, pp. 89–91, CBP.
37. A few months later, after returning to Washington, Barton wrote that the flying hospital changed locations "some eight or ten times" while she was with it. See CB to "Ladies of the Soldiers Aid Society, West Fitchburg, Mass.," January 26, 1865, B80, M63, pp. 89–91, CBP.
38. Parramore, "The Bartons of Bartonsville," pp. 22–40.
39. CB to Stephen Barton, March 1, 1862, B2, F4, AAS.
40. Stephen Barton to David Barton, October 23, 1864, B2, F6, AAS; CB to J. M. Barton, December 5, 1864, B2, F6, AAS.
41. Stephen Barton to David Barton, October 23, 1864, B2, F6, AAS; Stephen Barton to "My dear Friend," November 1, 1864, B2, F6, AAS; CB to J. M. Barton, December 5, 1864, B2, F6, AAS.
42. CB to J. M. Barton, December 5, 1864, B2, F6, AAS; Stephen Barton to David Barton, October 23, 1864, B2, F6, AAS.
43. CB to Elvira Stone, October 20, 1864, B14, R10, pp. 147–151, CBP; Pryor, *Clara Barton*, pp. 130–132; October 14, 1864, diary entry, B2, R1, CBP; William Barton, *The Life of Clara Barton*, 1:297.
44. October 12, 1864, diary entry, B2, R1, CBP; CB to Elvira Stone, October 20, 1864, B14, R10, pp. 147–151, CBP.
45. January 7, 1865, diary entry, B2, R1, CBP; CB to Judge Barton, December 4, 1864, Clara Barton Papers, American Antiquarian Society; Pryor, *Clara Barton*, p. 132. In November 1864, Stephen reported his feet and ankles "much swollen." Stephen Barton to Elvira Stone, November 1864, B14, R10, pp. 151–156, CBP.

46. "A Graphic and Excellent Letter from Clara Barton," undated newspaper clipping from the *New York Evening Express* found in B157, R110, p. 109, CBP.
47. Pryor, *Clara Barton*, pp. 74, 121, 142.
48. William Barton, *The Life of Clara Barton*, 1:294.
49. January 1, 1865, diary entry, B2, R1, CBP; Stephen Barton to Ada, etc., December 11, 1864, B2, F6, AAS; Voris, *A Citizen-Soldier's Civil War*, p. 235.
50. Stephen Barton to Ada, etc., December 11, 1864, B2, F6, AAS.
51. Voris, *A Citizen-Soldier's Civil War*, pp. 17, 235–238.
52. January 4–5, 1865, diary entries, B2, R1, CBP.
53. January 2, 3, and 7, 1865, diary entries, B2, R1, CBP. Of Kittinger, Barton wrote: "Although others of great worth may succeed him, no one can fully take the place of an old true and tried friend like D. K.—in all my trials for the two past years (almost) he has stood faithfully by me, endorsing every act, willing to cover, and forget every fault and resent every injury: Others may be all that could be expected under the circumstances but he has been more."
54. January 9–12, 1865, diary entries, B2, R1, CBP. Barton claimed Confederate pickets were just two hundred yards from the fort. In reality, they were at least six hundred yards away.
55. January 13–14, 1865, diary entries, B2, R1, CBP.
56. See January 12–14, 1865, diary entries, B2, R1, CBP.

CHAPTER 7. LATER YEARS

1. January 28–31, 1865, diary entries, B2, R1, CBP. Among other bills, Barton paid her landlord $65 to cover her rent from April 1864 to February 1865. Her landlord, Mr. Shaw, "objected to taking it," she wrote in her diary, "and would not count it. I left $65.00 for 9 mos @ 7 $ per month. paid for my Chronicle, 6.50." In addition to Mary Lincoln's reception, Barton went to a party celebrating the third anniversary of the United States Christian Commission, but the venue was so packed that she could not get in.
2. January 31 to February 1, 1865, diary entries, B2, R1, CBP.
3. January 31 to February 2, 1865, diary entries, B2, R1, CBP. Curtis had been wounded four times in the war and had lost his left eye in the assault on Fort Fisher. In 1891, he received the Medal of Honor for his actions in that battle.
4. February 10, 1865, diary entry, B2, R1, CBP. Years later, when residing in London, Barton occupied a house just a few blocks from Florence Nightingale. Although the two famous nurses corresponded briefly, they never met. "Remarkably similar in personality and aspiration," wrote historian Elizabeth Pryor, "neither could brook a competitor. Barton, who since 1862 had been continually called 'the Florence Nightingale of America,' noted with annoyance that no one was referring to Nightingale as the 'Clara Barton of Britain,' and was loath to put herself in a position requiring any sort of obsequiousness. Instead the two followed proper Victorian etiquette by exchanging a few notes, then literally taking to their beds to recover from the strain." Pryor, *Clara Barton*, p. 173.
5. February 10, 1865, diary entry, B2, R1, CBP.
6. February 12–14, 1865, diary entries, B2, R1, CBP. Oates, *A Woman of Valor*,

pp. 26–27, 294. Pryor, *Clara Barton*, p. 66. At that time tuberculosis went by the name of consumption.
7. February 10 and March 10, 1865, diary entries, B2, R1, CBP; Oates, *A Woman of Valor*, p. 303.
8. March 18, 1865, diary entry, B2, R2, CBP.
9. January 1, 1866, diary entry, B2, R2, CBP.
10. Paroled prisoners were released from confinement after agreeing not to take up arms again unless exchanged for a prisoner of the opposing army.
11. Ethan A. Hitchcock to CB, February 28, 1865, B80, M63, pp. 96–97, CBP; Henry Wilson to Abraham Lincoln, February 28, 1865, B80, M63, pp. 97–98, CBP.
12. Unidentified newspaper clipping in CB 1865 diary, B2, R2, p. 208, CBP.
13. Pryor, *Clara Barton*, p. 154; National Museum of Civil War Medicine website: http://www.civilwarmed.org/clara-bartons-missing-soldiers-office-2. Barton's office, located at 437 Seventh Street, N.W., was discovered in 1996. It is now open to the public under the auspices of the National Museum of Civil War Medicine.
14. B152, R107 ("Lectures and lecture notes, 1865–1868"), p. 92, CBP; "From Washington," *Cincinnati Commercial*, March 9, 1866, B80, R63, CBP. The prison's official name was Camp Sumter.
15. Andersonville National Historic Site website: https://www.nps.gov/ande/learn/historyculture/dorence_atwater.htm. A copy of Atwater's published register of Andersonville dead is in B79, R63, CBP.
16. *A List of Union Soldiers Buried at Andersonville*, p. iii.
17. Heitman, *Historical Register*, p. 474.
18. *OR* Series III, Vol. 5, p. 319; CB to "My dear friend," undated letter, B79, M63 (Andersonville prison, Miscellany, 1865 and undated), pp. 7–9, CBP; CB to Edwin Stanton, undated letter, B79, M63, pp. 39–44, CBP. Moore had received a brevet promotion to major on March 13, 1865. See Heitman, *Historical Register*, 1:474.
19. CB to "My dear friend," B79, M63 (Andersonville prison, Miscellany, 1865 and undated), p. 7; July 8, 1865, diary entry, B2, R1, CBP.
20. CB to "My dear friend," B79, M63 (Andersonville prison, Miscellany, 1865 and undated), pp. 7–14, CBP; CB to Edwin Stanton, undated letter, B79, M63, pp. 39–44, CBP; *A List of Union Soldiers Buried at Andersonville*, pp. iii, v.
21. CB to Edwin Stanton, undated letter, B79, M63, pp. 39–44, CBP.
22. CB to "My dear friend," B79, M63 (Andersonville prison, Miscellany, 1865 and undated), pp. 7–14, CBP; July 9–12, 1865, diary entries, B2, R1, CBP.
23. July 12, 1865, diary entry, B2, R1, CBP.
24. *OR* Series III, Vol. 5, pp. 319–320.
25. July 14–17, 1865, diary entries, B2, R1, CBP.
26. CB to "My dear friend," undated letter, Box 79, M63 (Andersonville prison, Miscellany, 1865 and undated), pp. 7–14, CBP; July 18, 1865, diary entry, B2, R1, CBP.
27. July 19, 1865, diary entry, B2, R1, CBP.
28. Ibid.
29. July 21, 1865, diary entry, B2, R1, CBP.
30. July 22, 1865, diary entry, B2, R1, CBP.

31. Ibid.
32. July 23, 1865, diary entry, B2, R1, CBP.
33. July 24, 1865, diary entry, B2, R1, CBP.
34. July 24–25, 1865, diary entries, B2, R1, CBP.
35. CB to Edwin Stanton, undated letter, B79, M63, pp. 39–44, CBP; July 25, 1865, diary entry, B2, R1, CBP.
36. CB to Edwin Stanton, undated letter, B79, M63, pp. 39–44, CBP.
37. July 25, 1865, diary entry, B2, R1, CBP.
38. CB to Edward H. Clement, B79, M63, pp. 9–12, CBP.
39. July 25, 1865, diary entry, B2, R1, CBP.
40. CB to Edwin Stanton, undated letter, B79, M63, pp. 39–44, CBP.
41. CB to Edward H. Clement, July 30, 1865, B79, M63, pp. 9–12, CBP. Moore agreed, writing: "Nothing has been destroyed. As our exhausted, emaciated, and enfeebled soldiers left it, so it stands to-day as a monument to an inhumanity unparalleled in the annals of war." See *OR* Series III, Vol. 5, p. 322.
42. CB to Mr. Brown, August 7, 1865, B79, M63, pp. 16–20, CBP.
43. Ibid. CB to "My dear friend," undated letter, B79, M63 (Andersonville prison, Miscellany, 1865 and undated), pp. 7–14, CBP; *OR* Series III, Vol. 5, p. 322.
44. CB to Edwin Stanton, undated letter, B79, M63, pp. 39–44, CBP.
45. Ibid.; CB to Mr. Brown, August 7, 1865, B79, M63, pp. 16–20, CBP.
46. CB to Edwin Stanton, undated letter, B79, M63, pp. 39–44, CBP; CB to Mr. Brown, August 7, 1865, B79, M63, pp. 16–20, CBP; *OR* Series III, Vol. 5, p. 322. "History of the Andersonville Prison," https://www.nps.gov/ande/learn/history culture/camp_sumter_history.htm.
47. *OR* Series III, Vol. 5, p. 320; CB to Edwin Stanton, undated letter, B79, M63, pp. 39–44, CBP; CB to Mr. Brown, August 7, 1865, B79, M63, pp. 16–20, CBP.
48. CB to Edwin Stanton, undated letter, B79, M63, pp. 39–44, CBP.
49. July 26 and August 8, 15–16, 1865, diary entries, B2, R1, CBP; CB to "My dear friend," undated letter, B79, M63 (Andersonville prison, Miscellany, 1865 and undated), pp. 7–14, CBP.
50. "Omnipresent and Omniscient: The Military Prison Career of Captain Henry Wirz," an article on the webpage of Andersonville National Historic Site: https://www.nps.gov/ande/learn/historyculture/captain_henry_wirz.htm.
51. CB to "My dear friend," undated letter, B79, M63 (Andersonville prison, Miscellany, 1865 and undated), pp. 7–14, CBP; CB to Mr. Brown, August 7, 1865, B79, M63, pp. 16-20, CBP.
52. "Clara Barton and Andersonville," an article on the webpage of Andersonville National Historic Site: https://www.nps.gov/ande/learn/historyculture/clara_barton.htm; Oates, *A Woman of Valor*, p. 330.
53. Wikipedia article on Champ Ferguson: https://en.wikipedia.org/wiki/ Champ _Ferguson; Wikipedia article on Henry Wirz: https://en.wikipedia.org/ wiki/Henry _Wirz. The only other man executed for wartime crimes was Champ Ferguson, a sadistic Confederate guerrilla who boasted of personally killing a hundred men.
54. Joel Griffin to CB, July 29, 1865, B79, M63 (Correspondence, Aug. 1864–Aug. 1911 and undated), pp. 7–8, CBP.

55. For an excellent summary of Joel Griffin's military service with the 15th Georgia Cavalry Battalion-Partisan Rangers, the 62nd Georgia Mounted Infantry, and the 8th Georgia Cavalry, see 62nd Georgia Regiment of Volunteers website: http://user.winbeam.com/~jagriffin/62nd.htm.
56. July 26–27, 1865, diary entries, B2, R1, CBP.
57. July 31 and August 2, 3, 4, 9, 10, and 12, 1864, diary entries, B2, R1, CBP.
58. July 26 and 31 and August 4 and 13, 1865, diary entries, B2, R1, CBP.
59. CB to "My dear friend," undated letter, B79, M63 (Andersonville prison, Miscellany, 1865 and undated), pp. 7–14, CBP; August 13, 1865, diary entry, B2, R1, CBP.
60. CB to "My dear friend," undated letter, B79, M63 (Andersonville prison, Miscellany, 1865 and undated), pp. 7–14, CBP; CB to Mr. Brown, August 7, 1865, B79, M63, pp. 16–20, CBP; August 1 and 7, 1865, diary entries, B2, R1, CBP.
61. CB to Edwin Stanton, undated letter, B79, M63, pp. 39–44, CBP.
62. August 4, 1865, diary entry, B2, R1, CBP.
63. CB to Edwin Stanton, undated letter, B79, M63, pp. 39–44, CBP; August 1, 1865, diary entry, B2, R1, CBP; *OR* Series III, Vol. 5, p. 321. Moore referred to Watts as a "letterer," someone who painted lettering on the headboards.
64. July 31 and August 1, 1865, diary entries, B2, R1, CBP.
65. August 14, 1865, diary entry, B2, R1, CBP.
66. August 15, 1865, diary entry, B2, R1, CBP.
67. August 16, 1865, diary entry, B2, R1, CBP.
68. August 17, 1865, diary entry, B2, R1, CBP. The author was unable to identify Mr. Walker.
69. August 22, 1865, diary entry, B2, R1, CBP. Copies of these letters appear in B79, M63 (Correspondence, Aug. 1864—Aug. 1911 and undated), B79, M63, pp. 13–15, CBP.
70. CB to Edwin Stanton, undated letter, B79, M63, pp. 39–44, CBP.
71. August 22, 1865, diary entry, B2, R1, CBP.
72. August 23, 1865, diary entry, B2, R1, CBP.
73. CB to Edwin Stanton, undated letter, B79, M63, pp. 39–44, CBP.
74. January 1, 1866, diary entry, B2, R2, CBP.
75. Heitman, *Historical Register*, 1:474.
76. September 30, 1865, diary entry, B2, R1, CBP; *Worcester Daily Spy*, June 26, 1866; Washington (DC) *National Republican*, September 26, 1865; *New York Herald*, September 19, 1865, and June 26, 1866; "Greatest Outrage of the War," *New York Citizen*, March 3 and 10, 1866; "Dorence Atwater," unidentified newspaper article. All the foregoing newspaper clippings appear in B80, R63, pp. 2–5, CBP.
77. "Dorence Atwater," https://en.wikipedia.org/wiki/Dorence_Atwater.
78. Pryor, *Clara Barton*, pp. 146–148. She also had a second clerk, Jules Golay. Both men lived with her at her Seventh Street residence.
79. "Dorence Atwater," *New York Citizen*, March 10, 1866, copy in B80, R63, p. 2, CBP; Pryor, *Clara Barton*, pp. 146–147.

80. For information on the salary Barton received from the Patent Office, see CB to D. P. Holloway, December 11, 1863, B1, R1, pp. 16–18, CBP; CB to Henry Wilson, April 7, 1864, B1, R1, pp. 52–55, CBP.
81. January 1, 1866, diary entry, B2, R2, CBP.
82. Pryor, *Clara Barton*, pp. 148–150; Oates, *A Woman of Valor*, p. 340; Lecture poster, B155, M109, p. 3, CBP; CB lecture records, B154, R109, p. 58, CBP; CB lecture schedule, B155, M109, p. 5, CBP; National Education Association, *Journal of Proceedings and Addresses*, p. 77.
83. Pryor, *Clara Barton*, pp. 160–161.
84. Ibid., pp. 175–189.
85. Ibid.; Barton, *The Life of Clara Barton*, 2:235.
86. "Veterans Meet," undated article in the *Worcester Daily Spy*; B155, R109, p. 47, CBP. Barton similarly wore her medals at American Red Cross functions. See Pryor, *Clara Barton*, pp. 271–272.
87. Pryor, *Clara Barton*, pp. 361, 366.
88. Barton, *The Life of Clara Barton*, 2:374–379; "Pneumonia Fatal to Clara Barton," unidentified newspaper clipping in B157, R110, CBP.
89. "Clara Barton," unidentified newspaper clipping in B162, R114, p. 21.
90. "The Founder of the American Red Cross," *Outlook*, April 20, 1912, copy in B162, R114, p. 12, CBP.
91. The buildings are the Clara Barton house in Glen Echo, Maryland; her birthplace in Oxford, Massachusetts; and her Missing Soldiers Office in Washington, D.C.

APPENDIX

The entire text of this speech may be found in the "Speeches and Writings File, 1849–1947; Speeches and lectures; War lectures, 1860s," B152, R107, pp. 208–221, CBP. It appears to be a copy of a handwritten speech now in the Special Collections of Smith College, Massachusetts. The Library of Congress's typescript can be found on line at its web site: http://www.loc.gov/resource/mss11973.107_0270_0490/?sp=208.

1. In June 1862, President Abraham Lincoln appointed Maj. Gen. John Pope to command the Army of Virginia, a force comprised of units defeated by "Stonewall" Jackson in the Shenandoah Valley. After checking the Army of the Potomac's advance on Richmond in the Seven Days battles, General Robert E. Lee dispatched Jackson with a force to "suppress" Pope. On August 9, Jackson fell on one corps of Pope's army, defeating it at Cedar Mountain. Lee then joined Jackson with the balance of the Confederate army and attacked Pope's main force along the banks of Bull Run, where Union and Confederate forces had first clashed back in July 1861. The Confederates again emerged victorious, driving the Federals back to their Washington, D.C., defenses. Of the 14,000 casualties in Pope's army, approximately 1,700 were killed on the field of battle. The rest were wounded, captured, or missing.
2. Records for Massachusetts and New Jersey troops show no one named Charley Hamilton being wounded at Second Manassas.
3. This paragraph, omitted in some transcriptions of the speech, was taken from a copy of the speech found in a folder entitled "War lectures, 1860s" in B152, R107,

pp. 103–104, CBP. The bracketed words were illegible in the original and were added by the editor.

4. "Gold Lace" refers to officers; "army blue" to the men in the ranks.

5. In her original typescript, Barton mistyped the word "murky" as "musky" and inadvertently left out the words "ran over our heads and mingled." These deficiencies do not appear in an earlier handwritten copy of the text that appears in a folder titled "Lectures and lecture notes, 1865–1868," in B152, R107, p. 220. In that manuscript, Barton put the time of the storm at 4 P.M. rather than 6 P.M.

6. After the Battle of Second Bull Run, Lee executed another turning movement in an effort to strike Pope's army as it retreated to Washington. On September 1, Jackson's Corps encountered the Union divisions of Isaac Stevens and Philip Kearny near the village of Chantilly. The Federals attacked Jackson amid a violent thunderstorm, and in the fighting that followed both Stevens and Kearny were killed. The action allowed the rest of Pope's army to escape to Washington. With Pope no longer a menace, Lee was free to carry the war into Maryland.

7. Barton exaggerates the proximity of the battle, which took place fully eight miles from Fairfax Station. She also misrepresents the goal of the Confederates, which was not to capture the field hospital at Fairfax Station but to destroy Pope's army.

8. Taken from James Hislop's poem, "A Cameronian Dream." For the full text of this poem, see Hood, *The Peerage of Poverty*, pp. 425–426.

9. *The Widow Bedott Papers*, by Frances Miriam Whitcher, was a popular satire on Victorian life. When the character Aunt Silly is offered a piece of chicken pie (not cabbage), she replies: "Well, I don't care if I dew take a leetle mite on't. I'm a great favoryte o' chicken pie—always thought 't was a delightful beverage." See Whitcher, *Widow Bedott,* p. 165.

10. A conical tent supported by a center pole.

11. Almira Fales. For additional information about Fales, see Chapter 1.

12. A surcingle is the belt that passes underneath the belly of a horse.

13. Here Barton lists Union forces that Lee and Jackson had vanquished earlier in the year. Major General Ambrose E. Burnside at this time led the Union army's Ninth Corps, which had just come up to Virginia from North Carolina. Major General John C. Frémont had been in command of the Mountain Department in West Virginia before being defeated by Maj. Gen. Richard S. Ewell at Cross Keys in the Shenandoah Valley. What Barton refers to here as the Army of the Peninsular was actually Maj. Gen. George B. McClellan's Army of the Potomac, which had suffered defeat at the gates of Richmond during the Peninsula Campaign.

14. Upon transferring to the Eastern Theater to take command of the newly created Army of Virginia, Maj. Gen. John Pope issued a bombastic address in which he claimed to "have come to you from the West, where we have always seen the backs of our enemies; from an army whose business it has been to seek the adversary, and to beat him when he was found; whose policy has been attack and not defense." *OR* 12(3):474.

15. The Peninsula Campaign, which began with the siege of Yorktown and concluded with the Battle of Malvern Hill, was a defeat for the Army of the Potomac.

16. Daniel H. Rucker (1812–1910) was still a colonel at the time. He would be appointed brigadier general of volunteers in May 1863 and breveted major general of volunteers in March 1865.
17. The foregoing portion of the text ("I was to ride 80 miles . . . sit down with four men") appears in Clara Barton's handwritten draft of the speech, now in the possession of the Sophia Smith Collection at Smith College, Massachusetts. It does not appear in Barton's typescript copy of the speech, on file in the Clara Barton Papers at the Library of Congress.
18. A large, heavy-duty trunk similar to later steamer trunks.
19. Major General Jesse L. Reno died at Fox's Gap, one of three South Mountain passes defended by the Confederates.
20. Frederick, Maryland.
21. Here Barton quotes scattered lines from John Greenleaf Whittier's poem "Barbara Frietchie."
22. A line from Thomas Moore's poem, "The Fire-Worshippers." See Moore, *Poetical Works*, p. 56. A footnote in the book identifies a kerna as the kind of trumpet "used by Tamerlane, the sound of which is described as uncommonly dreadful, and so loud as to be heard at the distance of several miles."
23. Taken from Sir Walter Scott's poem "The Lady of the Lake," Sixth Canto, Stanza XV. See Scott, *Complete Works*, 1:484.
24. Major General Joseph Hooker led the Army of the Potomac's First Corps, which opened the Battle of Antietam with an attack on the Confederate left.
25. This was the farm of Joseph Poffenberger, which stood just north of the North Woods.
26. The Poffenberger porch is far too narrow to hold four operating tables.
27. Generals Hooker, John Sedgwick, Napoleon J. T. Dana, George L. Hartsuff, and Joseph K. F. Mansfield each was a casualty of the battle. Sedgwick's wounding left Brig. Gen. Oliver O. Howard in command of the Second Division of the Second Corps, but he did not command the army's right wing.
28. The entrance to the Poffenberger cellar is on the opposite side of the house from the chimney.
29. A place of slaughter.
30. The entire text of this speech may be found in the "Speeches and Writings File, 1849–1947; Speeches and lectures; War lectures, 1860s," in Box 152, Reel 107, pp. 161–182, in the Clara Barton Papers at the Library of Congress in Washington, D.C. The Library of Congress has digitized the collection and it can be accessed at its web page: http://www.loc.gov/item/mss119730804. There are several versions of the speech, all virtually the same.
31. The teamster's full name was George Morton. See the memorandum section at the beginning of Barton's 1863 diary, B1, R1, p. 4, CBP.
32. Barton returned to Washington on December 31, 1862, following the Battle of Fredericksburg. It is unlikely her teamsters remained with her after that point.
33. Brigadier General Alfred Pleasonton commanded a division of cavalry in the Army of the Potomac's Right Grand Division.

34. Taken from "John Brown's Body," a Union army camp tune sometimes called "John Brown's Song." Julia Ward Howe later drafted new lyrics for the piece, which thereafter became famous as "The Battle Hymn of the Republic."
35. Major General Ambrose E. Burnside reluctantly took command of the Army of the Potomac on November 9, 1862.
36. The Rappahannock River flows past the city of Fredericksburg, Virginia.
37. Barton's reference here is to the tardy arrival of the pontoon bridges, which Burnside needed in order to cross the Rappahannock River.
38. Adapted from Reginald Vere's poem, "The Battle of Lansdown."
39. Major Generals Joseph Hooker, William B. Franklin, and Edwin V. Sumner commanded the Army of the Potomac's three grand divisions, each of which numbered approximately 35,000 men.
40. James Horace Lacy owned Chatham, a large colonial-era house situated on the left bank of the Rappahannock River, directly opposite Fredericksburg. Lacy, a major in the Confederate army, had acquired Chatham shortly before the war and was indeed present with the Confederate army at Fredericksburg. He later claimed to have entreated General Robert E. Lee to shell Chatham in the belief that Union officers were using it as a headquarters. According to Lacy, Lee refused because he had courted his wife there, a statement now discredited by historians. Barton was familiar with the plantation, having camped on the property during her previous visit to Fredericksburg in August 1862. See Lacy, "Lee at Fredericksburg," p. 606.
41. The struggle in town was far more obstinate than Barton describes. Confederate troops tenaciously defended Fredericksburg until sunset and then retired to Marye's Heights, half a mile west of town.
42. The Union army as a whole crossed the Rappahannock on December 12, one day after the street fighting that Barton describes. The heaviest fighting took place on December 13. At this point in her narrative, Barton inserted a lengthy poem, which has been excised from the present text.
43. Brigadier General Marsena R. Patrick.
44. A reference to Napoleon Bonaparte's wife, Josephine. Barton actually spelled the name "Iosiphine."
45. Barton added the foregoing phrase in earlier drafts of the speech.
46. An allusion to Lieutenant General Ulysses S. Grant.
47. The ridge adjoining Belle Plain rises to a height of 152 feet above sea level.
48. The Battle of the Wilderness, May 5–7, 1864, was fought in a tangled woodland fifteen miles west of Fredericksburg.
49. What Barton is trying to say is that fresh troops and supplies for the army traveled from Washington to Belle Plain by ship and that wounded men traveled from Fredericksburg to Belle Plain by wagon. At the landing the wounded soldiers were transferred from the wagons to the ships, which carried them back to Washington, while the supplies were taken from the ships and placed aboard the wagons, which carried them to the front.
50. Barton's diary indicates that she was still in Washington on May 8. Julia Wheelock, who accompanied Barton on her trip down the Potomac, noted that the ship arrived at Belle Plain on May 12. See Wheelock, *The Boys in White*, p. 187.

51. Planter's Hotel, at the northwest corner of William Street and Charles Street.
52. Secretary of War Edwin M. Stanton and possibly others.
53. Brigadier General Montgomery C. Meigs.
54. Barton returned to Fredericksburg on May 21, five days after the Quartermaster General's arrival.

Bibliography

MANUSCRIPTS

American Antiquarian Society, Worchester, Massachusetts
Clara Barton Papers
Edward M. Barton Papers
Andover-Harvard Theological Seminary, Harvard Divinity School, Cambridge, Massachusetts
Joseph Hamilton, "Clara Barton"
Boston Public Library, Boston, Massachusetts
Josiah F. Murphey, "Reminiscences"
Duke University, Durham, North Carolina
Mary Norton Papers
Fredericksburg and Spotsylvania County Battlefields Memorial National Military Park, Fredericksburg, Virginia
John J. Hennessy, 1860 map of Fredericksburg, Virginia
Wolcott P. Marsh letter
Edward K. Russell letter
National Archives and Records Administration, Washington, D.C.
John L. Brinton, "History of the Army of the Potomac from October 1, 1862, to December 20, 1862, with an account of the battle of Fredericksburg." Record Group 94, Entry 628, National Archives, Washington, D.C.
P. A. O'Connell, "Report of Medical Statement 9th Army Corps, Battle of Fredericksburg Va. Dec. 13th 1862," Record Group 94, Entry 544, A.C. Reg. No. 95
New York State Library, Albany, New York
Orsel Brown Papers
Gouverneur K. Warren Papers

Library of Congress, Washington, D.C.
Clara Barton Papers
Gouverneur K. Warren Papers
New Hampshire Historical Society, Concord, New Hampshire
George H. Chandler Papers
New Hampshire State Archives, Concord, New Hampshire
Executive Papers
Smith College, Northampton, Massachusetts
Clara Barton Papers, Sophia Smith Collection
University of Virginia
James L. Dunn Papers

NEWSPAPERS

Fitchburg (MA) *Sentinel*
Lowell (MA) *Daily Citizen and News*
Meadville (PA) *Crawford Journal*
New York Times
Philadelphia Sunday Morning Dispatch
Washington (DC) *Chronicle*
Worcester (MA) *National Aegis*

PUBLICATIONS

Abbott, John S. C. *History of Josephine*. New York: Harper & Brothers, 1852.

Adams, George Worthington. *Doctors in Blue: The Medical History of the Union Army in the Civil War*. New York: Henry Schuman, 1952.

Alexander, Edward P. *Military Memoirs of a Confederate: A Critical Narrative*. New York: Charles Scribner's Sons, 1907.

Alvey, Edward, Jr. *History of the Presbyterian Church of Fredericksburg, Virginia, 1808–1976*. Fredericksburg: Session of the Presbyterian Church, 1976.

The American Annual Cyclopaedia and Register of Important Events of the Year 1863. 3 vols. New York: Appleton & Company, 1864.

Annual Report of the Adjutant-General of the State of New York for the Year 1902. Serial No. 33. Albany: Argus Company, 1903.

A.S.B. "How Clara Barton Kept a Secret." *Woman's Journal*, February 24, 1883.

Bainbridge, Lucy S. "Three Pictures of Abraham Lincoln." *Outlook*, 118 (Jan.–April 1918), 244.

Barton, Clara. *The Story of My Childhood*. New York: Baker & Taylor, 1907.

Barton, William E. *The Life of Clara Barton: Founder of the American Red Cross*. 2 vols. Boston: Houghton Mifflin, 1922.

Bates, Samuel P. *History of Pennsylvania Volunteers, 1861–5*. 5 vols. Harrisburg: B. Singerly, 1869.

Bliss, Zenas R. "Types and Traditions of the Old Army." *Journal of the Military Service Institution of the United States*, 38 (May–June 1906), 516–529.

Boatner, Mark M. *The Civil War Dictionary*. New York: David McKay, 1988.

Bollet, Alfred J. *Civil War Medicine: Trials and Triumphs*. Tucson, Ariz.: Galen Press, 2002.

Brockett, Linus Pierpont. "Clara Harlowe Barton." *Appleton's Journal: A Magazine of General Literature*, 7 (February 24, 1872), 204–208.

———. *Lights and Shadows of the Great Rebellion: Or, The Camp, the Battle Field and Hospital*. Philadelphia: William Flint, n.d.

Brockett, Linus Pierpont and Mrs. Mary C. Vaughn. *Women's Work in the Civil War: A Record of Heroism, Patriotism and Patience*. Philadelphia: R. H. Curran, 1867.

Burton, Deloss S. "Spotsylvania: Letters from the Field: An Eyewitness," *Civil War Times Illustrated*, 22, no. 2 (April 1983), 22–26.

Carpenter, Francis B. *Six Months at the White House with Abraham Lincoln*. Bedford, Mass.: Applewood Books, 1866.

Dawes, Rufus R. *Service with the Sixth Wisconsin Volunteers*. Marietta, Ohio: E. R. Alderman & Sons, 1890.

Duncan, Louis C. *The Medical Department of the United States Army in the Civil War*. Gaithersburg, Md.: Butternut Press, 1985.

Dunn, James L. "Clara Barton," in Frank Moore, *Anecdotes, Poetry, and Incidents of the War: North and South*. New York: Printed for the Subscribers, 1866.

Dyer, Jonah F. *The Journal of a Civil War Surgeon*. Edited by Michael B. Chesson. Lincoln: University of Nebraska Press, 2003.

Emerson, William A. *Fitchburg, Massachusetts, Past and Present.* Fitchburg: Press of Blanchard & Brown, 1887.

Epler, Percy H. *The Life of Clara Barton.* New York: Macmillan, 1915.

Goss, Warren L. *Recollections of a Private.* New York: Thomas Y. Crowell, 1890.

Hanson, E. R. *Our Woman Workers: Biographical Sketches of Women Eminent in the Universalist Church for Literary, Philanthropic and Christian Work.* Chicago: Star and Covenant Office, 1884.

Harrison, Noel G. *Fredericksburg Civil War Sites, December 1862–April 1865.* 2 vols. Lynchburg: H. E. Howard, 1995.

Hart, Albert Bushnell. *The Romance of the Civil War.* New York: Macmillan, 1914.

Heitman, Francis B. *Historical Register and Dictionary of the United States Army, from Its Organization, September 29, 1789, to March 2, 1903.* 2 vols. Washington, D.C.: Government Printing Office, 1903.

Hood, Edwin P. *The Peerage of Poverty; or, Learners and Workers in Fields, Farms, and Factories.* London: S. W. Partridge & Co., n.d.

Howard, Victor B. *Religion and the Radical Republican Movement, 1860–1870.* Lexington: University Press of Kentucky, 1990.

Hurd, Daniel Hamilton. *Worcester County, Massachusetts, with Biographical Sketches of Many of Its Pioneers and Prominent Men.* 2 vols. Philadelphia: J. W. Lewis & Co., 1889.

Kerr, Paul B. *Civil War Surgeon: Biography of James Langstaff Dunn, MD.* Bloomington, Ind.: Authorhouse, 2005.

Krick, Robert K. *Civil War Weather in Virginia.* Tuscaloosa: University of Alabama Press, 2007.

Lacy, James H. "Lee at Fredericksburg." *Century Illustrated Monthly Magazine* 32, new series: vol. 10 (May to October 1886), 605–608.

Larcom, Lucy. "Clara Barton, the Founder of the Society of the Red Cross," in James Rudolph Garfield, ed., *Public Service.* Boston: Hall and Locke, 1911.

A List of the Union Soldiers Buried at Andersonville Copied from the Official Record in the Surgeon's Office at Andersonville. New York: Tribune Association, 1866.

Lord, Edward O., ed. *History of the Ninth Regiment New Hampshire Volunteers in the War of the Rebellion.* Concord, N.H.: Republican Press Association, 1895.

Lossing, Benson J. *Pictorial History of the Civil War in the United States of America.* 3 vols. Hartford, Conn.: Winter, 1866–68.

Massachusetts Soldiers, Sailors, and Marines in the Civil War. 8 vols. Norwood, Mass.: Norwood Press, 1931.

The Medical and Surgical History of the War of the Rebellion (1861–65). 6 vols. Washington, D.C.: Government Printing Office, 1875.

Miller, Francis T. *The Photographic History of the Civil War.* 10 vols. New York: Review of Reviews, 1912.

Moore, Frank. *Women of the War; Their Heroism and Self-Sacrifice.* Hartford, Conn.: S. S. Scranton, 1866.

Moore, Thomas. *The Poetical Works of Thomas Moore Complete in One Volume.* London: Longmans, Green, 1865.

Moss, Lemuel. *Annals of the United States Christian Commission.* Philadelphia: J. B. Lippincott, 1868.

National Education Association. *Journal of Proceedings and Addresses of the Forty-Fourth Annual Meeting Held at Asbury Park and Ocean Grove, New Jersey, July 3–7, 1905.* Winona, Minn.: National Education Association, 1905.

Nicolay, John G. and John Hay. *Abraham Lincoln: A History.* 10 vols. New York: Century, 1890.

Oates, Stephen B. *A Woman of Valor: Clara Barton and the Civil War.* New York: Free Press, 1994.

O'Reilly, Francis A. *The Fredericksburg Campaign: Winter War on the Rappahannock.* Baton Rouge: Louisiana State University Press, 2003.

Parramore, Thomas C. "The Bartons of Bartonsville." *North Carolina Historical Review* 51, no. 1 (Jan. 1974), 22–40.

Patrick, Marsena R. *Inside Lincoln's Army: The Diary of Marsena Rudolph Patrick, Provost Marshal General, Army of the Potomac.* Edited by David S. Sparks. New York: Thomas Yoseloff, 1964.

Pryor, Elizabeth B. *Clara Barton, Professional Angel*. Philadelphia: University of Pennsylvania Press, 1987.

Reed, William Howell. *Hospital Life in the Army of the Potomac*. Boston: William V. Spencer, 1866.

Register of Officers and Agents, Civil, Military, and Naval, in the Service of the United States, on the Thirtieth September, 1859; With the Names, Force, and Condition of All Ships and Vessels Belonging to the United States, and When and Where Built; Together with the Names and Compensation of All Printers in Any Way Employed by Congress, or Any Department or Officer of the Government. Washington, D.C.: William A. Harris, 1859.

Ross, Ishbel. *Angel of the Battlefield: The Life of Clara Barton*. New York: Harper & Brothers, 1956.

Ross, J., ed. *The Book of Scottish Poems: Ancient and Modern*. Edinburgh: Edinburgh Publishing, 1878.

Schouler, William. *A History of Massachusetts in the Civil War*. 2 vols. Boston: E. P. Dutton, 1871.

Schultz, Jane E. *This Birth Place of Souls: The Civil War Nursing Diary of Harriet Eaton*. New York: Oxford University Press, 2011.

Scott, Walter. *The Complete Works of Sir Walter Scott; With a Biography, and His Last Additions and Illustrations*. 7 vols. New York: Conner & Cooke, Franklin Buildings, 1833.

Smith, Adelaide W. *Reminiscences of an Army Nurse During the Civil War*. New York: Greaves, 1911.

Smith, Edward P. *Incidents Among Shot and Shell*. N.p.: Edgewood, 1868.

Smith, Stephen B. *Record of Service of Connecticut Men in the Army and Navy of the United States During the War of the Rebellion*. Hartford: Press of Case, Lockwood, and Brainerd, 1889.

Tower, Henry M. *Historical Sketches Relating to Spencer, Mass*. 2 vols. Spencer, Mass.: W. J. Heffernan—Spencer Leader Print, 1902.

Turino, Kenneth C., ed. *The Civil War Diary of Lieut. J. E. Hodgkins, 19th Massachusetts Volunteers, from August 11, 1862 to June 3, 1865*. Camden, Me.: Picton Press, n.d.

The United States Christian Commission for the Army and Navy: Works and Incidents. Third Annual Report. Philadelphia: n.p., 1865.

Voris, Alvin C. *A Citizen-Soldier's Civil War: The Letters of Brevet Major General Alvin C. Voris*. Ed. Jerome Mushkat. DeKalb: Northern Illinois University Press, 2002.

Walcott, Charles. *History of the Twenty-First Massachusetts Volunteers in the War for the Preservation of the Union 1861–1865 with Statistics of the War and of Rebel Prisons*. Boston: Houghton Mifflin, 1882.

War of the Rebellion: A Compilation of the Official Records of the Union and Confederate Armies. 128 vols. Washington, D.C.: Government Printing Office, 1880–1901.

Weymouth, A. B. *Memorial Sketch of Lieut. Edgar M. Newcomb of the Nineteenth Mass. Vols.* Malden, Mass.: Alvin G. Brown, 1883.

Wheelock, Julia S. *The Boys in White: The Experience of a Hospital Agent in and Around Washington*. New York: Lange and Hillman, 1870.

Whi[t]cher, Francis [*sic*] M. *The Widow Bedott Papers*. New York: J. C. Derby, 1856.

Willis, Henry A. *Fitchburg in the War of the Rebellion*. Fitchburg, Mass.: Stephen Shepley, 1866.

INTERNET RESOURCES

62nd Georgia Regiment of Volunteers http://user.winbeam.com/~jagriffin/62nd.htm.

Andersonville National Historic Site https://www.nps.gov/ande/learn/historyculture/clara_barton.htm. https://www.nps.gov/ande/learn/historyculture/dorence_atwater.htm. https://www.nps.gov/ande/learn/historyculture/camp_sumter_history.htm. https://www.nps.gov/ande/learn/historyculture/captain_henry_wirz.htm.

Dorence Atwater: https://en.wikipedia.org/wiki/Dorence_Atwater.

Clara Barton Papers, Library of Congress http://www.loc.gov/item/mss119730804.

Brager, Bruce L. "The City Point Explosion" https://www.militaryhistoryonline.com/civilwar/articles/citypoint.aspx.

Find a Grave (Archibald G. Shaver) http://www.findagrave.com/cgibin/fg.cgi?page=gr&GRid=8374076.

Champ Ferguson: https://en.wikipedia.org/wiki/Champ_Ferguson.

National Museum of Civil War Medicine: http://www.civilwarmed.org/clara-bartons-missing-soldiers-office-2.

National Museum of Health and Medicine: Dr. Daniel S. Lamb (Reeve 093786), https://www.flickr.com/photos/medicalmuseum/3300121774/.

Henry Wirz: https://en.wikipedia.org/wiki/Henry_Wirz.

Acknowledgments

This book could not have been written without the help of many kind individuals. Foremost among these are my former colleagues at Fredericksburg National Military Park, particularly Chief Historian John Hennessy, Cultural Resources Manager Eric Mink, and Green Springs Manager Noel Harrison. John helped me to identify people and places mentioned in Clara Barton's speech and produced a map of Civil War Fredericksburg that I used as the basis for one of the maps in this book. Noel pointed me toward potential Clara Barton sources, while Eric reviewed the manuscript and offered helpful suggestions toward its improvement. In addition, Historian Stephanie Gray of Antietam National Battlefield kindly shared with me her insights regarding Clara Barton at that battlefield.

Individuals outside the National Park Service also extended their help. Nancy Jahnig helped me track down Archibald Shaver's photograph, an image that Gerald K. Williamson generously shared with me. Dr. Eric W. Boyle of the National Museum of Health and Medicine kindly secured for me a copy of Daniel Lamb's image, while John McAnaw and Jenee Lindner shared with me their knowledge of Clara Barton's activities at Fairfax Station. Andrew Bourque assisted me during my visit to the American Antiquarian Society of Worcester, Massachusetts, and graciously copied for me dozens of pages from that institution's collection of Clara Barton Papers. Cartographer Hal Jespersen created four of the maps in this volume. The high quality of his work speaks for itself.

Finally, I wish to thank publisher Bruce H. Franklin, manuscript editor Noreen O'Connor-Abel, and the other members of the Westholme Publishing staff for making this book a reality.

Index

Page numbers followed by *ph* indicate an illustration or its caption. Those followed by *m* indicate a map.